ONE MAN
EXPECTANT FATHERHOOD

We haven't had sex for two weeks.

"Some women who've never had orgasms or a strong sex drive sometimes become very aroused and active during pregnancy," Francesca reads from one of our pregnancy guides. "Other women who've had a high sex drive prior to pregnancy lose some, if not all desire in the first trimester."

"The answer is B," I announce. To myself.

I find myself fantasizing about sex. Sex with a twenty-something college coed. Sex with a thirty-something actress. Sex with basically *any* woman I can imagine. I keep these thoughts to myself, locked away in an undetectable corner of my brain. In Francesca's heightened emotional state (the currently acceptable term for "unbalanced"), telling her I'm fantasizing about other women would cause undesired consequences, something involving ambulances and disability insurance.

"I'm sorry we're not having sex, Perry," says the clairvoyant.

"Francesca, I love you. I'm doing fine."

"You miss it, don't you?" She sets the bait. In a moment of clarity, I turn away from the lure.

"No, Francesca, I don't."

"You're sure?"

"Absolutely."

She knows I'm lying.

We turn out the lights, close our eyes and drift off to sleep.

I am surrounded by six eager sorority girls all named Kimmy. As they descend upon me, each removing a piece of my clothing, three cheerleaders also named Kimmy join the impending Roman orgy.

"This is going to be some night," I chuckle.

"Uh-huh," whispers Kimmy 4.

"Do you have health insurance?" asks Kimmy 7.

My Wife Is Pregnant
or
The End of the World as I Know It

My Wife Is Pregnant
or
The End of the World as I Know It

By

Perry Herman

First published by AuthorHouse 06/30/04

ISBN: 1-4184-7154-2 (e-book)
ISBN: 1-4184-5290-4 (Paperback)

Library of Congress Control Number: 2002095886

This book is printed on acid free paper.

Printed in the United States of America
Bloomington, IN

THIS BOOK IS DEDICATED TO MY WIFE, MY SON AND
MISTER FLUFFY.

Author's Note

While this book is based on actual events, I have taken some artistic liberties. Certain moments came entirely from my imagination. For example, Mister Fluffy, the talking pregnancy pillow, didn't really speak. Names have been changed to protect people's privacy. Finally, some passages present events that, in actuality, embody amalgams of true experiences.

My Wife Is Pregnant
or
The End of the World as I Know It

I'm lying in bed listening to Art Bell, the late-night talk show host with the latest on Area 51, alien invasions, and black helicopters. Tonight's topic: Remote Viewing. Accomplished remote viewers can mentally transport themselves to any part of the planet. Regular people like me can become Viewers–as long as we carefully study a three-cassette video course called *Remote Viewing: One, Two and Three*. (Available for two hundred and fifty dollars, tonight only.)

Frank, a remote viewer from Idaho, recounts how he recently solved a murder committed in Auckland, New Zealand. Someone had bludgeoned a bartender, but the local police could not find a suspect or motive.

"Through mental transportation," explains Frank, "I traveled from my three-car garage to the pub. It was closing time. All the patrons had left. I heard a scuffle. Then I saw it: a bearded man with a frozen ice block flew into a rage. The barkeep didn't know what hit him. One minute he's cleaning glasses, the next he's dead."

"Let me get this straight," says Art, "You actually saw the murder being committed?"

"That's right," proclaims Frank. "I gave the authorities a description of the killer. Next day the bartender's estranged half brother confessed to the crime."

"That's incredible. Just incredible."

"Perry?" My wife, Francesca, calls out in the dark.

"I'm listening to a remote viewer from Idaho."

"Come to the bathroom."

"He figured out who killed a bartender in New Zealand."

"Come to the bathroom," persists Francesca. An odd urgency colors her voice.

I climb out of bed. Back muscles tense the moment my warm feet touch the cold wooden floorboards. I plod down the hallway, squinting as I approach bright, harsh bathroom light.

"Quick!"

"Coming," I gurgle.

Francesca sits on the tile floor staring at a small, Popsicle-shaped object.

"Look!" she says.

"Two pink stripes," I observe. The words echo through my head, bouncing off every convolution, bone and lobe. Two pink stripes. Two pink stripes. Two pink stripes.

The first stripe is the test stripe. If it's pink, the test is accurate. It's pink. The second stripe is the hCG stripe. If it's pink, hCG is present. It's pink. hCG means the person taking the test is pregnant. Francesca just took the test. Francesca is pregnant. I'm pregnant. We're pregnant.

I should be jumping up and down with glee. That's how a husband is supposed to react when he sees two pink stripes. I am not jumping up and down. Francesca should be jumping up and down. That's how a wife is supposed to react when she sees two pink stripes. She's not jumping up and down. We are shocked. Our eyes meet in mutual disbelief.

Francesca is a survivor of stage two endometriosis, a disease that scars the uterus and, ultimately, renders a woman sterile. The surgeon who treated Francesca's condition told us our chances of being parents were small at best. From then on we had sex without contraception. Sometimes we had a "scare." I'd rush down to the nearby twenty-four hour mega-pharmacy and purchase a pregnancy test. I'd race home, Francesca would take the exam, and moments later would see one pink stripe. Not two. One.

We've become accustomed to the notion of a childless marriage. We've envisioned a future entirely focused on career and travel. We've planned to vigorously support Francesca's rapid rise through the corporate ranks. We've set our sights on sending my acting career through the stratosphere.

"What happens now?" I ask.

"We get a second opinion," she answers. Always the clear thinker.

The two of us stand before the medicine chest mirror. We consider our reflections in the glass. Francesca's beautiful skin. A pimple on my cheek.

Perry and Francesca. Husband and wife.

Perry and Francesca. Mom and Dad?

Outdated issues of *Consumer Reports* litter the bland waiting room. Beyond a door marked Enter, some unknown nurse extracts blood from Francesca's arm. Ten minutes stretch into twenty, then fifty. Finally she emerges.

"What did they do, take a gallon?"

Francesca doesn't hear my quip. Instead, she takes my hand and smiles softly. "I'm pregnant."

We hold each other.

I'm going to be a father.

Panic. Francesca remembers she had her hair colored on Saturday. According to one of the ten pregnancy books we bought yesterday, a big No-No along with Advil and refined sugar is hair dye.

"The chemical dye is absorbed through the scalp, into the bloodstream, and to the fetus. Although no side effects have been..." I stop reading. I can see Miss Clairol traveling through Francesca's blood stream and into the fetus. DNA strands become horribly tangled. The clock spins forward two years; my baby waves to me with three hands. In less than a month of pregnancy, we've blown it. The disdainful OB/GYN wagging her finger at us. Our parents, crestfallen.

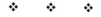

My therapist assures me Miss Clairol will not deform our baby.

My therapist assures me we will not be rendered bankrupt by our baby.

My therapist assures me we will make great parents and still be successful in our careers.

For some reason Career remains on par with Baby. I feel guilty harboring such thoughts. I know they are wrong but, apparently, I'm not alone. Everyone talks about the importance of having children, but when was the last time you saw a career-minded person bring an infant to an office meeting? Or to an audition?

We've already chosen names for our baby. We picked them three years ago. Roma, if it's a girl. Max, if it's a boy. Roma could be the cute tomboy, the girl who breaks all the boys' hearts as they, one by one, throw themselves at her feet, begging for just one sign of affection. Max could be the cute guy, the boy who follows in his dad's footsteps, pining for the cute brunette who doesn't know he exists. Maybe Max isn't a good name.

"Don't touch me," Francesca says in a playful, but serious manner.

We haven't had sex since we learned of our impending parenthood.

"You did this to me," proclaim her crossed arms. "You keep that thing away from me."

It's as if she believes we'll have a second child the moment we revisit intercourse. The other baby would secretly hide in some corner of Francesca's uterus, only to reveal itself moments after the birth of our first child.

"Congratulations, it's a boy!" the delivering doctor would say. "What's this?" A frown forms above the surgical mask.

I don't think it's scientifically possible to have an "on-deck" baby. But strangely, I don't want to have sex either. I'm already in deep enough.

I find myself ten years old again, plodding up a dirt trail, trying to keep pace with my father who walks ahead. He offers me a reassuring smile.

"It's not much farther," he promises.

Only his face is not my father's face. It's my face. And the ten-year-old is my ten-year-old. I cannot see the child's face. I cannot make out its sex. I cannot hear its voice.

I think of all the faded photographs of my dad holding me in his arms. I remember looking at those pictures and remarking wondrously, "My dad looks so young. I can't believe he was ever that young." My father was thirty-two when I was born. I'm thirty-two.

Nausea and fatigue have forced Francesca to do the unthinkable—take a sick day and watch videos. I offer my bedridden patient water and sneak a peak of "Washington Square," starring Jennifer Jason Leigh. I remember when I first fell in love with Ms. Leigh, a Saturday matinee of "Fast Times at Ridgemont High." I found her dark, mischievous eyes impossibly alluring. A half hour later I lost my innocence when she stripped naked and had sex with a slimy guy in a poolside cabana—an image forever burned into my adolescent brain. As "Washington Square" careens towards its desperate end, an intense passion overcomes Francesca and me. Our bodies intertwine, and soon we are making love as if it were the first time. Time disappears. I'm no longer sure where my body stops and hers begins. An hour passes. A blur. We lay on our backs exhausted. If this is pregnancy, I love it.

The Expectant Father's Guide forces me to face a stark reality: I know nothing about pregnancy and parenting.

"Why didn't they teach this in college?" I ask aloud.

Quiz me about Western European social thought, and I could go on for hours. Test me about gestation, and you'll see two very wide, blank eyes.

Francesca talks so quickly I haven't a clue what she's saying.

"And then this idiot tells me he doesn't know where he sent the promo discs. Can you believe that? What a jerk. I mean, my God! And then the developer on the manufacturing database, well he's a jerk too, and this morning I found myself drinking a vanilla milkshake. I hate vanilla. It's too sweet. You know I like chocolate. And so I force them to open the ice cream counter early because I need this ice cream—this milk shake—and then these people from my office see me drinking this shake at ten in the morning and this woman says, 'What are you, pregnant?' Do you think they can tell? Can you tell? Am I showing? I can't be showing yet, because if I'm showing, it'll screw everything up. I mean, people say, 'You should get pregnant.' But, if you tell them too soon, your career gets crushed. So, anyway, the guy still can't locate the promo discs—"

"What promo discs? Which guy?" I ask.

"The guy who didn't know where he sent the promo discs."

I wish I had popcorn. That would make this a movie and everything would be alright. But, I don't have popcorn, and this is real. My wife has lost her mind.

"We won't be able to give you a quote until late next week. We're really backed up. Everyone is," explains Sheri, my over-the-phone sales counselor.

I'm getting bids on new rain gutters. Just four months ago we bought our house "as is." I wish I'd looked up the phrase, "as is," in a real estate dictionary. That way I could have mentally prepared for life in the Money Vortex.

"Well," I exhale, "I guess there's not much to do except wait for—"

A raw, guttural sound rattles down the hallway. Francesca, half dressed for work, runs past me, her face frozen in a ghastly expression.

"Sir?" asks Sheri.

Francesca takes a sudden, jagged left turn into the bathroom. The door slams shut. The toilet seat crashes against porcelain. And then—The Sound. The sound that sends me straight back to freshman year. The sound I heard every weekend when the latest victim of alcohol poisoning careened into the bathroom and simultaneously ejected breakfast, lunch and dinner. Only it's eight in the morning. On a weekday. And Francesca hasn't been drinking.

"Oh my God!" I exclaim.

"Sir? Is everything alright?"

"Uh…"

"It sounds like someone is choking…"

"It's okay, it's just my wife."

"Sir?" My sales counselor is stunned by my callous disregard for Francesca's health.

"She's…" I can't say. No one can know. Not even a stranger. Not even Sheri, the rain gutter sales rep. That was the deal. "We went to a party last night. I guess she's not quite over it." Liquor. Always the best excuse.

"On a Tuesday night?" persists Sheri.

"Thanks so much." I slam the telephone handset into its cradle and rush to the bathroom.

Francesca lies prone on the floor. The sound of flushing water reverberates off the tiles. Wooosh. Wooosh. Wooosh.

"Are you okay?" I can't believe I just said that. Does she look okay? She's just vomited, she's writhing on the floor, and she's moaning.

"I can't believe you just said that," snaps Francesca, her eyes ice cold.

When a man says, "We're pregnant" or "I'm pregnant," he's lying. I'm not nauseous. Francesca is nauseous. I'm not curled up on the floor. Francesca is curled up on the floor. No matter how sensitive and enlightened I try to be during the next eight months, I will never know what it's like to be pregnant. *Thank God.*

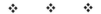

The comfort of my therapist's office is astounding: textured yellow walls, the furniture's soft cotton fabric. My stomach churns slowly, just as it has all week.

"I've been really edgy this week," I begin. "I'm second-guessing myself in auditions. It's like I doubt my ability to do what comes naturally to me. I know it has nothing to with the fact that we're pregnant…I mean…she's pregnant…because we've been really cool about it this week. So, it's, well, very confusing. I mean, I'm doing good work. All the casting directors have been really positive. And so, I know, objectively that is, that I'm still doing good work. But, there are these voices, and I'm not sure why they're there. Because I've really dealt with my whole performance anxiety thing and all. So, whatever. I mean. Well, what I'm saying is I've been edgy about my work, which is pissing me off because I've come so far with the whole anxiety thing this year. I mean, what do you think? Why do think I've been this way? Why am I this way now?"

"You're going to be a dad. That's why," answers my therapist.

"Because it's really strange. There's no reason why anything should be different. I should be more confident about my work than ever before. I mean, why? That's what I keep asking myself."

"You're going to be a dad. That's why," repeats my therapist.

"I mean, it could be that it's the end of the year, and I'm wondering if next year will be as successful. Or maybe, I don't know. What do you think?"

"You're going to be a dad. That's what."

"You think it's because I'm going to be a dad?"

"Uh-huh."

"I guess that makes sense."

"Uh-huh."

"Same time, next week?"

"Uh-huh."

I awake with a start.

"6:30 AM," says the Sony clock radio.

"Furniture. Must move. Furniture. Must move." The chant speeds through my head. My grandmother's piano will arrive Tuesday, and we still haven't made room for it.

Our house is already packed to the gills. The floors and walls explode with shelves, chairs and the Eight-Foot Crushed Velvet Couch. Years ago, a delivery truck arrived at Francesca's studio apartment with The Couch. The movers had to detach the behemoth's legs, just to avoid crushing the front door frame. Once inside, the green monster monopolized a third of the living area. We had to climb over an armrest, just to get to the kitchen.

The soon-to-arrive, instrument is mammoth—practically six feet by six feet. The thought of three burly men waiting impatiently for me to solve the space crisis is too much to bear. I awaken Francesca.

We stand in the living room, ready to solve the furniture challenge: Find a location for the piano without forcing a hulking, two-piece oak hutch, an over-sized glass coffee table, or The Couch into the garage.

Francesca thinks of a great idea. "Let's move the hutch out of the living room and into the baby room." Two weeks ago the Baby Room was Perry's Office.

"What about my desk? My *office* desk?"

"We'll move it into the breakfast nook," she replies, unfazed by my snippy attitude.

"Last time I checked," I fire back, "there was a dining table in the breakfast nook."

"We'll move it into the living room."

"The breakfast nook?"

"No, the table."

"Then where does the couch go?"

"We'll put it next to the French doors."

"That puts my computer cart in the baby room and my desk clear across the house in what, seconds ago, was the breakfast nook."

As I contemplate the piano's impeding size and mass, I realize the eighty-eight-key beast did not force me out of bed. The baby did. The reality of our baby. The reality that we must reconfigure our entire home to make room for Roma. Or Max. Or whoever shows up in eight months.

My life is turning upside down. Nothing is the same. My office desk is a changing table.

I have lost all bearings. I'm not sure which way is up or which way is down. I feel dizzy at times. My breath is shallow, my sleep fitful. Everything I've known is no more, and what is now is unknown. I am falling headlong into a deep, bottomless pit.

I look at my life. Everything appears as it has been. Our house still stands. Francesca goes to work every morning. My auditions and recordings continue. The sky remains hazy during the day and oddly luminescent through the night. I see my friends for lunch. I drive my car on the same freeways, which continue to be congested, stressful and inhuman.

Somewhere within Francesca's body, a life grows. Hands form. A heart evolves. A brain develops. A soul dawns. Somewhere within her. A child. A daughter. A son.

The old foundation crumbles away. Hopefully, something stronger, more durable will replace it. Something to give me strength on this new journey.

Next year, I will turn thirty-three and, soon after, I will be a Dad. It's a long way from college, a long way from childhood.

Yesterday a teenaged girl called me "Sir." I rush to the bathroom mirror and examine my hair for hints of gray.

The UPS man delivers a huge package from my mother. Inside is my childhood wrapped in newspaper: picture books, dolls and model cars. If I didn't know better, my mother already knows Francesca is pregnant. I burrow through crayon drawings of people, animals and space ships and arrive at a book called *Mean Max,* its illustrations instantly familiar. The objects somehow attest to my parents' awesome devotion, the countless hours they spent ensuring my future. I'm struck by how much they gave me. I'm amazed by how hard they worked to make me what I am today.

What a strange voyage, parenthood. Years of deeply challenging work and then, when your child is finally self-sufficient, he leaves you. If you've done your job well, he graces you with an occasional phone call or, in the rarest of occasions, an actual, hand-written letter. If you've failed, he never leaves, a permanent houseguest.

Fatherhood. It still strikes me as a surreal concept. Here I am in Hollywood, the nexus of eternal youth, a place where, like everyone else, I expected to be eternally twenty-six, single and edgy.

I'm sitting in a doctor's waiting room while Francesca dutifully completes a New Patient Form: Insurance Number. Work Phone Number. Person to Contact in Case Of Emergency. A young boy in a gray school uniform plays with small plastic pirates and their brown plastic galleon.

A nurse dressed in a teddy bear print blouse calls our name and leads us to an examination room.

"The doctor will be with you next," she says with a reassuring smile.

A cursory review of the room leads me to a three-inch, black and white television monitor, a computer keyboard, and a video recorder. I am thunderstruck. I am staring at a sonogram machine, the thing that makes black and white fetus pictures, the pictures our pregnant friends proudly display on their refrigerators. Francesca is thinking the same thoughts. She looks like a doe staring into oncoming headlights. The room is silent. We regard each other for a moment, as if meeting for the first time.

"Who's this guy who knocked me up?" her clenched mouth demands.

"Who's this woman who seduced me into becoming a dad?" fires back my furrowed brow.

Somehow sitting in this room, next to the video recorder, increases the reality of our situation fourfold. It's like looking at four pregnancy test kits and seeing two pink stripes on each one. It's like looking at eight pink stripes. Even in this surreal moment, I can still multiply.

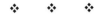

Thirty minutes pass. Apparently, "The doctor will be with you next" means "The doctor will see you some time today." I begin to wonder if there really *is* a doctor in the office. Maybe the whole place is a front for an insurance fraud scam. Maybe the nurse isn't really a nurse. Maybe we should leave while we still can.

The door opens. A tall, lanky man enters. He wears the requisite doctor costume: white coat with stethoscope. He looks authentic.

"I'm Doctor Braintree." He leads us into another room, his office. Diplomas of every kind adorn the walls. I decide the seals and signatures are legitimate. Doctor Braintree is, in fact, a genuine doctor.

Thick-framed plastic glasses rest on every flat surface of the room. One pair lays on the doctor's desk, another on a shelf, and a third on a file cabinet. A life-sized, wooden golden retriever sits next to us, ready to come alive at any moment.

"Nice dog," I say.

"Yes, as you can see, he's very well trained."

A joke. Our physician has a sense of humor.

"Do you have any questions?" he asks without emotion.

"How do you feel about cesareans?" I ask. He gives us a thorough, scientific response.

"How many babies have you delivered?" Francesca asks.

"Over five thousand," is his answer. I figure that makes him reasonably qualified to deliver our child.

Francesca takes a breath. Here comes the big one. "How do you feel about abortion?"

Francesca and I have talked about this question. If tests show our baby has severe birth defects or Francesca's life is in danger, we will abort the fetus. That's it. That's how we feel.

"I don't perform abortions," he replies without a hint of judgment. "But, I will refer my patients if such a decision is made."

The doctor tells us only one Los Angeles hospital is certified to perform second trimester abortions. I find this stunning. If America's second largest city has only one, there must be thousands of cities with none.

"What's the risk of miscarriage?" continues Francesca. A lot of our friends have had miscarriages.

"About one in six during the first trimester. But, if the fetus looks good in early sonograms, the odds for a miscarriage drop dramatically."

"When do we do the first sonogram?" I ask.

"Right now." He says in his usual, matter-of-fact tone.

The teddy bear clad nurse ferries us back to the examination room. She activates the machine while Francesca undresses and covers herself in a quilted, paper smock. The three-inch monitor ignites. On it appears the familiar geometric shape we've seen outlining all of our friends' refrigerator pictures. It looks like the profile of an oddly sliced piece of apple-pie. Various numbers and letters appear on the left and right margins of the screen.

The doctor puts gel on a long, plastic probe. Francesca gasps. I gasp. Our initial survey of the room overlooked this troubling gizmo. It looks unseemly. It looks imposing. To put it another way, it looks like a giant dildo. There, I said it.

"Is that going in…" Francesca asks cautiously.

"Yes, but I promise you, it's painless."

They all say that. Doctor's should be banned from ever saying, "It's painless."

The nurse offers me a chair. She's afraid I'm going to faint, not an unreasonable concern considering my sudden dizziness. I sit down. Francesca looks at me. I look at her. We stare into the screen.

"You see that?" the doctor asks.

I see squiggly lines, shadows and light spots.

"That's the yoke. At this early stage, we're not much different than chickens." Only a few rungs of deoxyribose nucleic acid separate my child from becoming a rooster.

"Now," he continues, "tell me what that is."

I look closely at the screen. I see it. It's a rhythmic pattern. A tiny dot turns black then white. If I were looking through a high powered telescope, I'd say it was a pulsar. The spot turns light. Then dark. Light. Then dark.

"Its heart?" I guess.

"Bingo."

Its heart. I'm watching its heart beat.

Suddenly everything is one hundred times more real than the first pregnancy test. It's like looking at one hundred pregnancy test kits and seeing two pink stripes on each one. It's like looking at two hundred pink stripes. You get the idea.

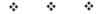

I peer inside a bulging plastic bag, an unexpected parting gift from the teddy bear nurse. Turning it upside down unleashes a torrent of objects: magazines, video cassettes and pamphlets.

Baby Magazine. Your complimentary copy!

Getting ready for baby? How to make all the right choices. BabysRUs. The Baby Superstore.

The Welcome Addition Club. Similac Infant Formulas.

Stork Avenue. America's Favorite Birth Announcement Company.

Pampers.

Evenflo.

Johnson & Johnson.

Huggies.

BabyCenter.com.

Aprica.

This isn't just a sack packed with promotional items. This is our official passport to a new consumer world. Today Corporate America christens us double-income, married, expectant parents living in a major metropolitan center. Thousands of databases across the United States simultaneously add our names to whirring hard drives. Automated printers and packagers start tons of direct mail on their way to our mailbox. Marketing specialists plot to make us customers for life. The nation's businesses wait breathlessly for us to slide our Visa card's magnetic strip through an electronic debit machine. They count the seconds until we complete our first baby-centric, web-based secure transaction.

We haven't had sex for two weeks.

"Some women who've never had orgasms or a strong sex drive sometimes become very aroused and active during pregnancy," Francesca reads from one of our pregnancy guides. "Other women who've had a high sex drive prior to pregnancy lose some, if not all desire in the first trimester."

"The answer is B," I announce. To myself.

I find myself fantasizing about sex. Sex with a twenty-something college coed. Sex with a thirty-something actress. Sex with basically *any* woman I can imagine. I keep these thoughts to myself, locked away in an undetectable corner of my brain. In Francesca's heightened emotional state (the currently acceptable term for "unbalanced"), telling her I'm fantasizing about other women would cause undesired consequences, something involving ambulances and disability insurance.

"I'm sorry we're not having sex, Perry," says the clairvoyant.

"Francesca, I love you. I'm doing fine."

"You miss it, don't you?" She sets the bait. In a moment of clarity, I turn away from the lure.

"No, Francesca, I don't."

"You're sure?"

"Absolutely."

She knows I'm lying.

We turn out the lights, close our eyes and drift off to sleep.

I am surrounded by six eager sorority girls all named Kimmy. As they descend upon me, each removing a piece of my clothing, three cheerleaders also named Kimmy join the impending Roman orgy.

"This is going to be some night," I chuckle.

"Uh-huh," whispers Kimmy 4.

"Do you have health insurance?" asks Kimmy 7.

My cousin Ralph and I finish a great Chinese lunch.

"You have time for a short walk?" I ask, still relishing the memories of sizzling rice soup.

Ralph checks his watch. "Sure."

We exit the restaurant. The sky is crystalline blue. November days in Los Angeles make you forget about its chronic smog.

"I'll put my backpack away before we start," I say.

We head over to my car. Ralph stands next to me. I open the trunk. There, in plain view, is a bag bursting with baby food samples. I shut the trunk. No one is to know. That's the plan. I check Ralph's face for any sign of recognition. I see none.

"I guess I'll just hold onto the backpack," I proclaim. "After all, my pager's in it."

Another brush with danger.

"Are my breasts getting bigger?"

"Huh?"

The clock radio reads 11:30 PM.

"Are my breasts getting bigger?"

I reach for the switch to my reading lamp. I find it. Bright white light cuts through the tranquil darkness. Francesca lies wide-awake. If there were ceiling tiles above us, she would be counting them.

I curiously regard her breasts, hidden underneath her favorite blue pajama top. "No, they don't look bigger," I say.

It's true, they look just like they did when I first met her. I also know, even if they are larger, I should still say, "No."

"Am I showing?" Francesca asks as she inspects her abdominal area.

"No, Francesca, you're not showing." I know this is a sensitive topic. "You're less than two months pregnant. You can't even begin to show for another four weeks." At least that's what the baby books say.

"I look okay?" she asks. Her face is so cute. Every day she looks prettier and prettier.

"You look beautiful," I say.

She smiles.

"God, I'm so tired," she exhales.

I almost say, "I know," but I know that I don't. I have absolutely no idea what she's feeling. I've actually lost weight in the past few weeks. I've felt awake, even buoyant—except, of course, during my occasional panic attacks.

Tonight, I realize it's my turn to be strong for Francesca and, remarkably, I feel solid. Tonight, I'm excited about being a father. Tonight, I am relishing the next seven months. I hold Francesca in my arms.

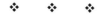

"We can't see you guys today," says my friend, David, in a pained voice.

"If you want to talk, I'm here," I say.

He sighs deeply. "Thanks."

I can tell David and Emily are in the midst of a horrible argument. The fluctuating voice and tense silences tell me they're hurling accusations at each other, accusations they're already regretting. They have two children. Two boys. A one-and-a-half-year-old and a three-month-old. They have plenty of money for a live-in nanny, Baby-Gap outfits and a shiny new Dodge Caravan SE, but their wealth cannot insulate them from the perils of parenthood. These are our closest friends. We have held their babies. We are Aunt Francesca and Uncle Perry to their children.

My friend calls again, "We're okay now. Sorry about canceling everything."

"You sound better."

"How 'bout dinner?"

Francesca and I listen to Alanis Morrisette as we battle The Ten. In Los Angeles, freeways are a constant, malevolent presence. They are our perpetual foes. Each of us has an intimate, painful relationship with these endless roadways. Every day we curse The Ten. Every day we bargain with The Four-O-Five. Every day we surrender to The One-O-One.

I'm glad we'll be seeing our friends today. Ever since we moved out of our old neighborhood, where they still live, we've made a point of getting together every Saturday. On one Saturday David and I take care of the kids while the wives enjoy a movie. The following week the women stay home, and we see a film. Every Saturday with the kids is an intense preview of my fatherhood future.

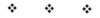

Francesca and I ride in the Dodge Caravan SE's back seats. David and Emily sit in front, constantly craning their heads back to monitor their boys' chaotic activities in Row 2, Seats A and B. The minivan is awe-inspiring: digital dashboard, leather seats, double sliding doors and a ten CD changer.

Bliss has returned to the family. The oldest boy smiles at his drooling, newborn brother.

"When we get back to the house, I want to show you something on the net," David tells me excitedly.

"What?" snips Emily.

"It'll just take five minutes," her husband replies defensively.

"Fine, just go and abandon the kids, why don't you?"

We wave goodbye. Our friends recede into the distance. Francesca and I squirm in our seats. We think the same thoughts.

"I don't want kids ruining our relationship," Francesca breaks the silence.

We both know our friends' marriage is strong, but we see the threat: screaming kids, two careers, and sleep deprivation. It can all lead to short tempers, jealousy and anger.

"It doesn't have to," I say hopefully.

"No, it doesn't have to," repeats Francesca aloud, as if saying the words again will make them more believable.

Traffic signs crawl past us.

"What if, each night, only one of us is responsible for dealing with the baby?" I suggest. "That way one of us will always have a good night's sleep, and no one will get overly tired."

"That's good." Francesca likes this tact.

Emboldened, I continue. "And if I have a big audition or gig the next day, you'll be on duty the night before, and if you have a big meeting the next day, I'll take care of everything. We'll be flexible. We'll work together."

Francesca brightens. "The person who's on duty could sleep in the baby's room. That way the other person could get uninterrupted sleep."

"What if we both have important appointments the next day?" I ask. "What do we do then?"

Silence.

Towering, stainless steel office buildings glisten in the distance.

"Well, then…" Francesca reaches for a solution. "We'll do something different."

"Right," I concur enthusiastically. "Something different." Our moment of reverie dissolves into a sudden, brief *poof*.

A rattling eighteen-wheeler spews thick, black diesel exhaust into the tea colored sky.

"I want our child to be comfortable with being independent. Even at age two I was very independent," declares Francesca.

"I think child care after the sixth month would be good. Our baby would get used to being apart from us and learn to feel secure on its own," I add.

"I don't want us to get a nanny."

"We're not going to spoil this kid."

We're on a roll.

We pull into our driveway. We're exhausted. Time has accelerated somehow. Our delivery date doesn't seem very far off. We have lots to discuss. We have lots to explore. We're going to be parents. More than ever, it's all so real.

Thanksgiving: Turkey, Pilgrims and unfortunate Indians.

My brother, Daniel, and his wife, Kate, have just arrived from wintry Boston to celebrate the holiday with us. Crisp air pierces our bodies as we sit around a flimsy, white plastic patio table. Francesca suggests I open a very nice bottle of champagne to welcome our arrivals. I oblige, sending a cork skyward.

I pour champagne for everyone except Francesca. As the bubbly flows, I sense the impending danger of this impromptu fete. An incredible bottle of champagne and, yet, someone declines to drink. In a soft drink situation, "No, thank you" generates nothing more than a pleasant nod. In an alcohol situation, minds race. "Is she an alcoholic?" "Is she being a prig?" "Oh my God, is she *pregnant*?" I wish Francesca had suggested a different beverage, something like Mr. Pibb. No one gets curious when you pass up a chance to drink Mr. Pibb.

"Aren't you going to have some, Francesca?" asks Kate innocently. The danger no longer feels impending. Now it's real and immediate.

"No, I'm fine." Francesca makes a point of relishing her lemon-lime water.

"But, it's really good," continues Kate, unaware of the havoc she is reaping.

A moment passes. My brother continues on about something or other. Kate pauses to regard Francesca. Francesca turns away. Her porcelain colored cheeks morph into crimson red flags.

"She knows," say Francesca's desperate, hazel eyes.

"I know," say Kate's apologetic, blue eyes.

It's obvious Kate had no desire to uncover our deepest secret. Uncovering deep secrets is generally not the thing to do when you're a brand new sister-in-law. My brother's lips continue to move. I hear nothing, but it's clear he has no idea what's happening. The cat, whichever cat that is, has just left the bag. I inhale deeply. My lungs defend themselves from a sudden rush of cold air. The bronchioles freeze. I sputter and cough. Nothing to do but confess. The cuffs are on. The chase has ended.

"You figured it out," I say with a smile.

"Figured what out?" my brother asks.

"Francesca is pregnant." There. I said it. Out loud. Francesca's face is completely red. I can't tell where her lips stop and the rest of her face begins. My brother regards me with total surprise and pleasure. He smiles in a way I've never before seen. The smile radiates love and compassion.

"This is so great!" he says. He can barely contain himself.

"Yup," says Francesca, "I'm pregnant."

"Congratulations," cheers Kate.

I feel relaxed beyond my wildest dreams. Our most important secret made public. For some reason, there isn't a tense muscle in my body. I notice my champagne glass is empty.

"How did that happen?" I ponder as I pour myself another one.

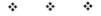

Disneyland. The happiest place on earth. If waiting in line makes you happy.

Francesca, Kate, Daniel and I approach the Star Cruiser 3000. We've been waiting more than an hour to ride Star Tours. This is our favorite ride. A brightly illuminated sign warns us of the risks we face: *Persons with back, neck or other muscle problems should not ride. Expectant mothers should not ride.*

Francesca waves goodbye. As we enter the Star Cruiser 3000 and prepare for our journey to Endor, she heads back to Earth via a door marked Exit.

Indiana Jones and the Temple Of Doom. *Expectant Mothers should not ride.*

Splash Mountain. *Expectant Mothers should not ride.*

Space Mountain. *Expectant Mothers should not ride.*

Rocket Rods. *Expectant Mothers should not ride.*

Peter Pan. Thank god for Fantasyland.

Two days after Turkey. Churning stomachs and unbridled shopping. I ease the car into a narrow space. Other disgruntled autos honk in disgust.

"That was mine!" blares a monolithic Lincoln Navigator.

I hate shopping malls during the Christmas season. I hate the noise. I hate the food courts. I especially hate the insipid, ever-repeating Yuletide standards.

A country version of "Jingle Bells" rebounds off escalators and storefronts. Muslims, Buddhists and Jews cringe. *Dashing through the snow, y'all! On a one horse open sleigh, Yee-haw!* A banjo solo sends the outcasts into hopeless despair.

"I need new clothes," announces Francesca.

"Sure," I reply off-handedly.

"You don't understand the situation." Francesca grabs my hand. "None of my clothes fit. My jeans are so tight I can't breath. People at work will notice something's up if I don't buy new clothes. I need new clothes. I hate these jeans. *I hate them.* They make my hips look a mile wide."

Francesca paces outside Pregnancy Fashions and surveys passing shoppers. No familiar faces. The coast is clear. She scurries inside. We sift through a mass of bland merchandise.

Giant, shapeless coats hang on one side. Giant, shapeless dresses hang on the other.

Francesca and I regain our composure in an overly bright food court. Two unfortunate teenagers working at a hot dog stand suffer the humiliation of their official uniforms: shorts, tank top and a beanie—all striped red, yellow, blue and white. They look like defective Popsicles churning vats of lemonade.

"There are lots of other places," I say reassuringly. "Let's go somewhere more up-market. I want you to have clothes that make you feel comfortable. Who cares what it costs?" I'm learning.

We find a Limited. Francesca likes the Limited's European feel. A hypnotic, synthesized rendition of *We Wish You a Merry Christmas* echoes left and right. A bubbly salesgirl approaches us. Her nametag says, "Jenny."

"Do you need some help?" she asks as she pulses to the Christmas groove.

"I'm pregnant!" blurts Francesca.

"Congratulations!" applauds Gyrating Jenny.

Francesca models one piece of clothing after another. She slips into elastic waist pants and lycra stretch shirts. She sports baggy sweaters and elastic skirts. Each wardrobe elicits a careful evaluation in an unforgiving, floor to ceiling mirror. With each outfit her spirits rise or fall.

An hour of anguish and elation ends well. Francesca thanks Jenny, the twirling sales counselor, and exits the Limited with two bulging shopping bags.

❖ 2 ❖

Francesca lies next to the now familiar three-inch, black and white monitor. Doctor Braintree, our country-style practitioner, prepares the sonogram probe and embarks on the examination. I stare at the screen, anxious to see how much the fetus has grown. A silhouette appears, a faint white outline. I survey the screen for a key landmark: the tiny, pulsing heart. The probe moves back and forth. The flashing black and white sphere eludes the monitor's radiating sound waves. The examination stops.

"I'm so sorry."

Two masked orderlies wheel Francesca's gurney down a linoleum hallway.

"I'm so scared," says my wife.

"I love you," is all I can muster.

Francesca's feet disappear behind flip-flopping metal doors. Flip flop. Flip flop. Flip flop.

Outdated magazines. The click, click, click of a sterile wall clock. Time slows to an excruciating crawl.

"The procedure was successful." Doctor Braintree puts his arm around my shoulder. "I'm so sorry."

Tears fall from my cheek and splatter on the beige floor below.

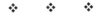

I steer the Maxima into a restaurant parking lot dominated by a large, illuminated House of Pies sign, spinning above a towering metal pole.

We choose a window booth and stare into our menus. I order a giant, messy hamburger filled with mayonnaise and pickles. Francesca chooses onion rings and a large chocolate milk shake. We hold hands across the table. Francesca sobs quietly. Tears well from my eyes.

"Things will get better," our waitress offers kindly.

My mother's uncanny timing strikes again.

"How are you doing?" she asks warmly.

I cannot answer the question.

"Are you and Francesca alright? Did you have a fight?"

"No, Mom." I struggle to contain my emotions.

"What is it, Perry?"

"Francesca was pregnant. We lost the baby. We just got back from the hospital."

"I'm so sorry."

I am twelve years old. I am hiding under my bed sheets, unable to face the world. My mother's soothing words cascade over me. For the first time in days, I believe the pain will eventually stop.

"If you want to talk, I'm here."

"Thanks, Mom."

"I love you, Perry."

"I love you, too."

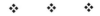

"Francesca was pregnant. We lost the fetus." I tell the painful story over and over as our friends, one by one, call to ask why Francesca was in the hospital. "Was she sick?" "Is she okay now?" "What happened?" With each repeat of the terrible truth, our friends, one by one, offer the same consolation: "At least you know you can get pregnant." Always said with compassion. Always impossible to hear without collapsing into sadness. Only David responds differently: "I'm so sorry, Perry." No silver lining. No reassuring thought. Nothing. Emily miscarried a year earlier. David understands. There is nothing to say.

A uniformed valet hands me a ticket while another carries our bags to the lobby. A white stucco interior welcomes us to a much needed getaway weekend.

A waiter seats us by a gurgling fountain and offers us crisp, white menus.

"Anything to drink?" asks the starched server.

"7 and 7," Francesca's terse response.

"Vodka Collins," I add. I sense trouble. I check Francesca's eyes. They swirl with accusation. "What?"

"Do you have any idea how I'm feeling these days?"

"Okay, I guess."

"Well, I'm not." Francesca stares straight through me. "You never ask me how I'm doing."

"I ask you about work all the time."

"That's not how I'm doing. That's work. That's not me. That's not my life. That's not us."

"Okay. Well, tell me then, how are you doing?"

"I don't feel like talking to you. I am so angry with you." In one breath Francesca finishes her drink and orders another. I can feel other patrons staring at us.

"Francesca," I try another tact. "This is your birthday weekend. You should be having fun. Let's work this through."

"Why does our relationship always have to be in serious trouble before you realize we need to talk?"

My stomach drops a floor. "What do you mean *serious*?"

"Did you know I find myself looking at other men, wondering what it would be like to date them?"

"Are you seeing someone?"

"Did you know a guy at work asked me out?"

My intestines hit the basement. "Are you having an affair?"

"What difference would it make to you? When was the last time we had sex?"

The eyes of strangers zero in on us, on me. Judging. Evaluating. Criticizing.

"Francesca, I love you. I care about you. How you're feeling."

"You sure have a crappy way of showing it."

"Please, tell me how you're feeling. I want to know. I'm interested."

"I don't feel like talking, alright? I'm tired. Let's just eat dinner."

Pasta Primavera. Sparkling water. Freshly baked bread. Silence. The bill.

I trail ten feet behind my wife as we wend our way towards our room and the pain its emptiness will bring. The click of the room's double lock reminds me of something David told me: "Be prepared for a rough period. It happens after a miscarriage. It's brutal."

A sleepless night. A lifeless breakfast. An argument in the middle of a street. Francesca storming out of a store. Me storming out of a store. Another sleepless night. Excellent scrambled eggs. Apologies. Hand holding. Kisses. Laughter. Understanding. Love.

I hand two dollars to a grinning hotel valet. I steer our car onto a bustling street of shops and cafes.

"I love you, Francesca."

"I love you, too."

Togos, our favorite sandwich shop.

I await a Number 20, a small-tuna-on-rye-with-light-dressing. Just as my mouth opens wide to receive the moist albacore, I notice a glare in Francesca's eyes. I am back at the hotel about to relive the Nightmare Dinner. I feel myself sinking into a deep pool of quicksand.

"You never focus on my feelings!" Francesca looks away. "You never talk about me. We're always talking about you."

I feel my blood temperature rise from a moderate 98.6 to a rolling boil. I find myself hovering outside my body watching me throw a medium iced tea across the restaurant. I hear myself scream, "I am not going through this bullshit again! You are crazy! You know that? You are CRAZY!"

I am lying in bed listening to a disembodied talk show host discuss the United Nations' secret agenda.

"Perry?"

"Some guy is explaining how the UN is taking over the world."

"Come to the bathroom."

"He says they have a secret base in Nevada."

"Perry, come to the bathroom."

I climb out of bed. Back muscles tense the moment my warm feet touch the cold wooden floorboards. I plod down the hallway, squinting as I approach bright, harsh bathroom light.

"Quick!"

"Coming," I gurgle.

Francesca sits on the tile floor staring at a small, Popsicle-shaped object.

"Look," she says.

"Two pink stripes," I observe. Two pink stripes. Two pink stripes.

❖ 3 ❖

The clock radio announces the first news of the day: violence in the Middle East, the NASDAQ's latest movements and, most importantly, box office earnings for the latest feel-good movie.

Francesca's arms wrap around my waist. She kisses me on the neck. A laugh. A smile. A twinkle.

"How'd I get so lucky?" she asks.

"Well, it all started fifteen years ago..."

I watch her apply eye shadow, slip into a smartly cut pinstripe suit, and battle with pantyhose, jewelry and hair rollers. The daily ritual for the modern American, upwardly mobile woman.

"Am I fat?"

"Pregnant, but not fat," I reassure her.

The professional woman must not be discovered too early in pregnancy. If the secret is revealed precipitously, the career mysteriously sidetracks. A female executive must spring the news no earlier than the four month mark, immediately broadcast her desire to find a nanny, and talk excitedly about returning to work only a few weeks after delivery. Her peers will do the math and conclude the two months lost to maternity leave aren't problematic enough to merit her replacement.

In the midst of sliding a black, high-heel shoe onto her right foot, Francesca loses balance. An outstretched arm and a nearby bedpost save her from an unceremonious collision with the hardwood floor.

"Morning sickness," she grunts.

"I'll get the soda water and crackers." We're old pros.

"I just need to rest a moment." Francesca lies prone on the bed. Seconds later she stands and tests her equilibrium. Notebook computer around one shoulder, handbag around the other, Francesca clatters down the driveway.

The car backs out into the street. Francesca waves. Taillights disappear around a corner. A pregnancy test awaits.

I dress and make my daily pilgrimage to the neighborhood coffee shop. As I head past a bustling nursery school, I imagine myself bounding up to the front door, meeting my child, giving her a hug and asking how her day was.

One decaffeinated coffee consumed and one morning paper read, I retrace my morning walk.

I launch my home office and check phone mail.

A disembodied female voice greets me: "First new message sent today at 9:43 AM."

A more familiar voice follows, Francesca on her car phone. "I'm driving back to work, and…We're pregnant…I love you. Congratulations. And, uh, let's hope…three months what does that make it?…So I guess in August we'll find out if this is gonna…this is gonna take. I hope it does. I love you. Bye."

"Message saved," reports my voice mail mistress.

Lunch with David, father of two.

A palpable panic courses through my veins.

"I was just in San Francisco, and I saw all these thirty-something types driving around in Z4 convertibles. And, well, they're all creating these start-up companies, and I keep thinking to myself—what kind of equity business am I building? I mean, as an actor, I can only control so much. Ultimately, my economic future is in the hands of some casting director or producer. My fate is held hostage by another person's whims."

David shoots me an odd, bemused look.

"Sure, things are okay now," I continue, "but what about in six months? What about a year? In this business you're up one day and down the next."

We finish lunch and walk through the surrounding neighborhood past a fabric mart, a gas station and an auto supply store.

"So, I've been working on a screenplay idea I've got." Thoughts gush from my mouth. "It's about these two guys, one's broke, the other's a computer programmer who hates his work."

After a half-hour or so, we climb into David's car, baby seat in the back.

"I feel like the clock is ticking. I feel like there's so much I could become. So much potential. Sometimes I feel like I still haven't found what I'm looking for." I've just quoted U2.

David calmly guides his sedan past tree lined streets.

"Francesca's career is clear. Every day she has a structure. Every day she moves towards a specific goal. She can quantitatively measure her growth. Me? Who knows? How can anyone in this crazy place know?"

We park in a shaded space out front of David's house. Emily stands on the doorstep holding Allen, their eldest son. Allen waves hello to his father.

"Perry," says David, "you're gonna be a great dad. Your kid isn't going to starve. Your career isn't going to end the moment your child is born. It's going to be the greatest adventure of your life."

"Thanks."

"Anytime."

Saturday morning. The regular complement of birds chirps outside. The unhappy dogs living in the upper canyon growl and whine. I roll to my left and find myself face to face with a sleeping Francesca, her body kept warm by thick flannel pajamas covered with pictures of bacon, eggs, hot coffee and pancakes. I quietly crawl out of bed, making sure not to wake her. All I can think of is breakfast.

Francesca returns from a flower cutting class.

"They had a contest, and I came in second."

She's sixteen again. She produces a beautiful floral arrangement. Stark white and pink flowers create a symmetric pattern framed by green leaves.

"I came in second!" she repeats.

Francesca rarely allows herself the luxury of a hobby. But, recently something has shifted. Her intensity has eased. She's begun to return home from work before eight. Saturday and Sunday afternoons at the office are but a memory.

"Let's go!" commands my wife.

Francesca's intensity hasn't eased at all. It has simply shifted from the office to our home. Suddenly every outstanding house project must be resolved today. This morning. Now. IKEA calls.

IKEA presents the greatest known threat to a healthy marriage. Everything about this self-service furniture store conspires to undermine a couple's mutual sense of trust and respect. The store lures customers into its cheerful yellow and blue showroom with the promise of beautiful European design, reasonable prices, and simple, at-home assembly. It's the simple at-home assembly that proves fatal. Building on past IKEA experience, we avoid the standard pitfalls. We check all the parts before leaving the store and, as usual, find many to be the wrong color and damaged. After replacing the defective items, we carry the unassembled LUMPENPOCK shelves to our car. IKEA assigns unpronounceable Swedish names to all of its furniture. You might find yourself buying a ZERKINPLINK mirror, an AUGENSTOCK couch, or an OOGLEMIT rocking chair. I wonder if the huge flat cardboard box containing the LUMPENPOCK will fit in our trunk.

Once home, we lay all the shelf parts out on the living room floor. We carefully examine the easy, step-by-step instructions featuring confusing diagrams and helpful tips in Swedish.

"We're going to do this together," I proclaim. Danger lurks in every corner of the room. "This will be simple and easy."

Inexplicably, the process proceeds quickly and painlessly. The shelves' outer frame assembles in less than an hour. Building on our positive momentum, we delve into the easy-click drawers.

"I need a mallet," says Francesca. The easy-click drawers aren't clicking easily.

Somehow I posses the presence of mind to avoid offering "helpful" suggestions. That's how the IKEA Syndrome begins. Husband questions wife's choice of mallet. Wife chastises husband for being a control freak. Distrust blooms. Husband and wife retain divorce attorneys.

Like a nurse handing a scalpel to a skilled surgeon, I pass the tool, saying only, "Mallet."

"Screwdriver," requests the furniture physician.

"Screwdriver." I pass a hefty Philips' head.

"Hammer."

"Hammer." I offer the tool handle-first.

A drawer clicks.

"Alright." The doctor inhales deeply. "I'm going to install the first drawer."

Francesca slides the drawer into the shelving frame. She jiggles it left, then right hoping to connect it to a drawer guide. The attempt fails.

"God dammit," exclaims the normally cool practitioner.

"What? What is it?" I inquire, even though I already know what's coming. It happens every time. At the most painful moment, the instant the point-of-no-return has passed, something goes terribly wrong.

"All the bolts are in backwards."

The simple, easy-to-read instructional drawings exact their expected revenge.

"Let's stop," suggests Francesca.

"What?" I gasp in disbelief. This is the moment when we blame each other for reading the diagrams incorrectly. This is when I hit the shelving frame with my fist. This is when the LUMPENPOCK becomes a metaphor for our entire, doomed relationship.

"Let's make some hot chocolate, watch a movie and go to bed." Francesca abandons the cluttered living room floor in favor of our bedroom.

"Right behind you." The sense of empowerment is almost too much to bear.

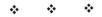

"Perry. Are you awake?"

I'm in a plush, red velvet chamber. Three naked supermodels gyrate to a provocative, tribal beat.

"Perry?"

"Perry?" inquires one of the supermodels whom I recognize from a Victoria's Secret catalog.

"Are you awake?"

The supermodel's face grows fuzzy and, in its place, my wife's beautiful face appears.

"Perry."

"Huh?" The only vocabulary currently available in my head.

"I can't sleep. My lower back hurts." Francesca's face is full of anxiety. "Is it normal to have back pain?"

I sit up, attempting to find vertical.

"Why do I feel so much pain?"

"It sounds pretty normal to me," I say. "All sorts of changes are happening around your uterus. It's bound to cause lower muscle pain." Another tidbit from our baby book library.

"I can't sleep."

"Let's listen to talk radio. That usually does the trick."

"I'm sorry I woke you up."

"I'm glad you did."

I turn on the bedside clock radio.

"Mental telepathy is the future of global law enforcement," exclaims an excited woman.

"Let me make sure I understand what you're saying," says Art. "Does that mean policemen might, someday, not have to patrol the streets to fight crime?"

"That's right," the caller replies assuredly. "They will be able to stay in their offices and simply scan the streets with their brainwaves."

"I love you." Francesca's words disappear into a snore.

Once again America's fringe lulls us to sleep.

"I'm afraid my career will end the moment the baby is born."

Francesca and I eat lunch at our local café. Francesca navigates a Tuna Salad on Focaccia. Spinach salad sits before me.

Francesca and I have an untraditional arrangement. She's the regular paycheck, and I'm the lotto ticket. Her consistent income enables us to pay the bills and sleep at night. My big hits pay for copper pipes and room remodels.

When the baby is born, Francesca will return to her office, and I will be the primary parent. I will continue to audition and work, but my life will be much more of a balancing act.

"I'm worried I'll be consumed by the parenting and drop out of an industry that has a one-day memory. I'm afraid I'll come back to my agents and they'll ask for ID."

"I know, Perry. I know."

I realize how deeply I trust Francesca. I know she loves the artist in me and will do anything to protect it. I know we'll find creative solutions to make acting classes, rehearsals and jobs still possible.

"The key," she continues, "is to find someone who can cover for a few hours here and there. Maybe a grad student. Maybe a local daycare center."

My salad's spinach leaves aren't cut small enough. I feel like a dinosaur chewing giant fronds off a prehistoric tree.

"How about some tuna?" offers Francesca.

Joy fills our car. The LUMPENPOCK shelves are finished. They reluctantly surrendered only moments ago.

I steer the car towards a retirement party for one of Francesca's coworkers. After a quarter century of loyal service, he's been forced out by a team of twenty-something management consultants. Consultants believe they will never be middle age, downsizing targets. Revenge is sweet.

As we merge onto the freeway, Francesca gazes out her window. I know this look.

"What's wrong?" I ask.

"I'm scared."

"Scared of what?"

"Going to the hospital. Of having another D and C."

A mile-high SUV swerves in front of us. Its tire flaps sport metallic silhouettes of naked women.

"I'm afraid of waking up in the recovery room, still under the anesthesia and hearing all the other patients cry and moan."

I've never undergone surgery. I've never come out of anesthesia.

"It's so scary. You're awake, but you can't move anything. You can hear the nurses complaining about some doctor, but you can't respond. You're totally vulnerable. Totally out of control. I don't want to go through that again. Ever."

There's nothing for me to say. I know this is a "listening" moment. I hold Francesca's hand and speed towards Burbank.

"Perry? Are you awake?"

I'm lying on a beach with four swimsuit models. Tropical breezes blow gently. Palm trees sway.

"Perry?"

"Perry?" asks Juliet, the French one with green eyes. I sit up and lean towards her.

"Are you awake?" asks Francesca, the pregnant one with hazel eyes.

"Yes, I'm awake."

"My back hurts, and I can't sleep."

The clock radio crackles to life.

"I've got an implant in my left pinky. It looks like a common wood splinter, but it's actually made of unknown polymers."

"Have any scientists examined the device?"

"No, Art. For some reason no one will return my calls."

Mike Myers pushes his latest film on the morning news. He's not much older than I. He's an established movie star. What am I? An unknown voiceover actor with nothing in development. A person who has never appeared in *People* magazine's *Star Tracks*. My lack of underachievement overwhelms me.

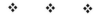

Francesca awakens with severe intestinal pain. She clutches her stomach, careens into the bathroom, and slams the bathroom door behind her. A cacophony of sounds seep through the keyhole: a lingering moan, water ricocheting off a cast iron bathtub, a toilet flush, the deafening roar of a hair blower.

A half-hour later she emerges. The office beckons.

"If I don't make the ship date for this week's album release," Francesca says to no one in particular, "there will be hell to pay."

"No auditions today," I whine from underneath the bed covers. "No work for two weeks." Hearing no response to my woes, I emerge from a mound of pillows to survey the landscape. My eyes locate a frowning Francesca. Her forehead creases. Her jaw tightens. I can see the doghouse. I can see myself in the doghouse. I think about apologizing immediately. I consider telling Francesca I'm a jackass for complaining about anything. I can stay at home. I can do whatever I want. I live the freelance life. She just finished vomiting and lamenting about her deadline. But I've already uttered the words. It's too late. I brace for the worst.

"You never do anything around here. Part of your job is to do house things. Then maybe we could spend a weekend at a museum instead of installing curtains. God, I'd love to stay home." She stomps down the hallway. "Pretty soon I won't be able to bend over. Then what happens? It's always the same thing with us. I'm always moving forward, and you're always holding us back. All you think about is your career. What about me? What about devoting a day to Francesca? Why don't you do house projects? There's so much stuff we need to do before the baby comes. 'Cause, once it's here, there won't be time for projects. None. Why don't you deal with the garage? It's a disaster. We need to organize it if we're ever going to get the house clean. What about your office? It looks like a mess. You notice how our friends' houses are neat and ordered? How do you think that happens? Do you think little elves magically appear in the middle of the night and organize their stuff?"

It's worse than I expected. The doghouse starts to look like an exotic resort in the Bahamas.

"Why don't you go to IKEA and finish the shelves in your office? Get the extra drawers you need. God, I wish I didn't have to go to work. I'd love to stay home. Really I would."

We stand on our front door stoop. Our next door neighbor walks past us. She senses the tension between us. The ultimate American humiliation. The secret is out. Soon everyone will know the Herman's had a fight.

"I wish, just once, you'd make us your top priority." Francesca climbs into the Miata and backs out of the driveway. "Call me on my cell," she grunts.

I call Francesca on the cell.

"I love you," she says, her words warped by a defective digital signal.

"I'm cleaning out the garage," I reply.

A blue recycling bin overflows with collapsed cardboard boxes and glass bottles. Damaged luggage, paint cans, and an old tire fill a voluminous black garbage can. I have conquered the garage.

I admire the expanse of empty concrete floor before me. I revel in neatly organized shelves and the total absence of cobwebs. For the first time I can actually park a car in the garage.

I wonder why I waited so long to do something so satisfying.

Birds on Franklin, a restaurant located across the street from a looming complex of buildings. Once a hotel. Now something else. Actors and people who look like actors saunter about, drink coffee and smoke cigarettes. Hot Los Angeles sun burns through a thick layer of carbon monoxide. I gulp down an iced tea and wave to Will.

Will. Probably the wisest friend I have. He's lived a lot. Sitting with Will realigns me. He's like a personal guide who's always a few steps ahead of me. He lets me know everything's going to be all right.

I tell Will about my current depression. I tell him work has slowed. I tell him everything except that I'm an expectant father.

Francesca and I have developed an odd sort of agreement. We tell someone we're pregnant only if Francesca feels it's *right*. The definition of *right* is nebulous at best. So far we've told her mother. But not her dad. We broke the news to her brother, but we haven't told my parents. The logic eludes me.

Will talks about a recent audition. I talk about Francesca's long work hours.

There's something very calming about having lunch with a gaggle of actors and writers who, like me, are all unemployed. Tourists visiting Hollywood must all ask the same questions: "Doesn't anyone work here?" "Is everyone a millionaire?" "Are all these actors living on the edge?" I know the answers. We all do. But we've pledged not to tell. Instead, we focus our attention on developing a façade of assurance based upon nothing but dreams and perseverance.

"You're gonna be alright," Will tells me. "You're a pretty together person."

I want to tell my parents we're pregnant. Maybe the time will soon be *right*.

"I'm in this giant high rise building filled with kids. I get in an elevator, and it starts to rise. Higher and higher it goes. Finally it stops. The doors open, and I'm on the top floor. I look out the window and discover the building is being engulfed by water. The water line rises and rises until the entire skyscraper drowns in water. It's totally submerged. There's no way out."

"Wow," I say.

"What do you think it means?" Francesca asks.

"That you feel incredibly overwhelmed by the prospect of a baby. That you're not sure you can handle motherhood and your fourteen-hour-a-day job. That you could drown in the awesome amount of responsibility you will face," I think to myself.

"It means you're very thirsty," I say aloud.

"Really?"

"Would you like me to get you a glass of water?"

"That sounds great."

I'm learning.

A rousing chorus of birds, dogs and a lost helicopter wake me. I hop out of bed and head for the bathroom. I shave, shower and dress for an industrious day at home. I feel the drive to create a nest for our coming addition. Delivery Day doesn't seem far off. I want us to be ready. My age-old desire to linger, to keep things as they've been, has vanished. I bound into the kitchen and prepare breakfast for Francesca: a multi-vitamin, orange juice, high-fiber cereal with milk, and a not-yet-ripe banana. Francesca's bananas must be green.

I poke my head into the bedroom. "Good morning, Sunshine!"

Francesca's eyes open slightly. "Sleepy," she says in a gurgle.

"It's a beautiful day. I've made breakfast for you. It's your favorite."

Francesca's eyes close. She rolls on her side and falls fast asleep.

Leaf blowers and rousing music emanate from adjoining properties. Rick, the window man, parks his black Nissan pickup truck in our driveway. He fishes through a toolbox and begins cutting replacement glass for the baby room. Francesca, the unstoppable, wildly industrious, high-powered executive, snores loudly, her body wrapped in a thick comforter.

My arm and shoulder muscles ache. Three hours of hacking away at vines, crabgrass and roots have taken their toll.

For months the back yard has been our personal Jurassic Park. When I was a child, ancient ruins fascinated me. I tried to guess how long it would take for a building to fall apart and become completely engulfed in vegetation. One thousand years seemed like a reasonable estimate. I was wrong. Home ownership offers a different answer: ninety days.

"Hi," Francesca calls from the patio. She sports flower print shorts and her favorite Maine sweatshirt, the green one with a giant red lobster embroidered on the front. "I'm exhausted."

"You've been working hard these past weeks, anyone would be wiped-out."

"I'm really tired. Really tired."

"We've got a long weekend in front of us. All you have to do is relax."

Francesca eyes the dirt beds I've just cleared. The gears begin to turn.

"Let's get trees," she declares suddenly.

Total exhaustion. Tree purchase. The connection eludes me. I proceed with caution. "Are you sure?" I ask.

"Let's go. Now."

"We need to replace the bushes out front with drought resistant plants," Francesca says within minutes of arrival at the nursery.

"I thought you just wanted to get trees."

"I do but we need plants, too." My wife leads us to a giant selection of desert vegetation and vacillates between Rose of Sharon and aloe vera. She takes two of each and places them in a cart she's just grabbed. "We need flowers for the patio area." The pregnant landscaper bolts toward rows and rows of cosmos, sunflowers and daisies. Soon our cart overflows with greens, yellows and blues.

"I have to go," Francesca abruptly announces.

"What?"

"I have to leave. Right now."

"We haven't gotten to the trees. That's why you wanted to come here in the first place."

"We're leaving."

Francesca struggles out of our car, limps towards the front door, disappears into the bedroom and falls fast asleep.

I remember reading something about the first trimester. Something about unbelievable exhaustion, an inability to make choices, and an immediate, overwhelming compulsion to finish every house project imaginable.

The backyard looks twice as large. A pile of brush towers into the sky. Sweat beads down every inch of my body.

Francesca sleeps soundly, her thoughts ensconced in some vivid dream world. I pray she's not back in the water-logged skyscraper, frantically searching for the nearest emergency exit.

I tell my father we're pregnant.

"That's wonderful," he cheers.

"You're going to be a grandfather!"

Silence clogs our phone connection. Being a grandfather means my father is no longer thirty-five.

"I still feel so young," he says. "Just yesterday, I held you in my arms."

"Let's have sex," suggests Francesca.

"Okay," I respond stupidly.

Men are dogs. The instant a woman suggests sex a man undergoes an immediate transformation. His tongue wags. His penis enlarges. His eyes widen. All he thinks of is intercourse.

Within seconds we're entwined. And within seconds I'm on top of her, ready for the big moment.

"You're not enjoying this, are you?" I observe.

"What do you think?"

"I just went for it, didn't I?" The it, being IT.

Francesca's arms cross. "There's this thing women enjoy. It's called foreplay."

It's an odd thing to be sexually reviled by the woman who carries your baby. It's not something I ever considered. I never wondered, "What would it be like to strike-out with my pregnant wife? What would that be like?" Now I know.

"Hello?" my mother answers the phone sleepily.

I check my watch. I can't believe it's only seven in the morning.

"Sorry, Mom. I didn't realize how early it is."

"Is something the matter?"

"No. I have some news."

"You're pregnant?" My mother, always one step ahead.

"Yes."

"I knew it!"

My mom really wants a granddaughter. She wants a cute, hell-raising granddaughter.

We've been invited to the Magic Castle for brunch. It's a members-only club for magicians. We're meeting a recently divorced friend and her new beau. She's very excited about the new boyfriend. In fact, they've already discussed having children.

We arrive at the castle and find ourselves face to face with Bill. Bill looks to be fifty-two years old. His unsettling grin betrays his true thoughts: *I'm banging a woman who could be my daughter. What do you think about that?*

During brunch, he tells me his penis is three times larger than our friend's ex-husband's penis. "Mine is so big, I can't even get it in all the way," he whispers in my ear.

"We're going to go to Italy for a two week bike ride," our friend glows. "We'll stay at five-star hotels and eat gourmet meals the whole way."

Bill explains how he converted junk bonds into real estate and BMWs. His college age kids sit across from us. They scan the dining hall, hoping to find a replacement for their pathetic father.

I've never felt so thankful Francesca and I were born in the same decade. I am grateful we both grew up on Depeche Mode and that neither of us was alive when "Rebel Without a Cause" premiered.

Our friend waves goodbye as her grinning, sunglasses-shrouded boyfriend powers his midnight black 745i out of the valet driveway.

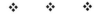

I park the Maxima out front of Don and Jim's home. Francesca is apprehensive. Our friends have an incredible wine collection, and they love to drink it. They also insist on sharing it. Only Francesca can't drink, and no one outside the immediate family can know The Secret. According to Francesca, the time still isn't yet *right*.

We navigate a flight of Spanish tile stairs, circle around to the back of the house and grab a chair next to the brand new pool; its waterfall, glistening blue tile, and adjoining Jacuzzi lull us into reverie.

"Wine?" offers Jim.

"Thanks," I say.

"Francesca?"

"How about some sparkling water?" she asks awkwardly.

"Sure…" Jim's a bit lost. Hollywood Hills. California sun. Brand new pool. Sparkling water?

Don finishes barbecuing chicken and vegetables on his outdoor DCS gas grill. My mouth waters in anticipation.

Jim emerges from the wine cellar with an incredible bottle of Chardonnay and ceremoniously approaches our candlelit dining table. "One for Francesca…" He pours the liquid gold into a glistening, crystal flute.

"Do you have any more sparkling water?" Francesca squirms in her chair.

"Sure…" Jim replies uncomfortably. He casts Don a questioning look. Don discretely shrugs his shoulders.

"I have something to tell you." Francesca takes a breath.

My eyes widen.

"You can't tell anyone," she pleads.

"Promise," assures Don.

"What is it?" asks Jim, expecting the worst.

Francesca takes a deep breath. Jim and Don brace for the news.

"I'm pregnant!" she blurts.

Don and Jim let out a huge, simultaneous sigh of relief.

"We were so worried," exclaims Don.

"We thought you were dying," says Jim.

"Why didn't you tell us?" asks Don.

We spend the next three hours gorging on great food and conversation.

"Can you drive?" I ask Francesca as we wave goodbye to our hosts.

"Why?" she asks.

"I'm drunk."

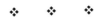

We decide to pay David and Emily a surprise visit. We find them at a waning Memorial Day block party, a few doors down from their home. Their two-year-old, covered in face and body paint, says, "Hello." He wears a tie-dye T-shirt and a huge smile. We help carry a grill, a Radio Flyer wagon and some chairs back to the house. Soon everyone assembles around the dining table.

"If there's one thing I can recommend," advises David, "have help from Day One...maybe you guys are different from us, but we couldn't have done it without a nanny. It's just too much."

I find myself thinking about money. About how much we'll need to pay for all the baby expenses. I think about how slow my business has been this year. I think about mortgage payments, property tax and how much pressure Francesca feels as the regular paycheck.

"You okay?" asks David.

"Huh?" I say. "Oh, yeah. Fine."

David knows I'm lying.

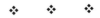

A woman stands at a bus stop, an infant strapped to her body. The baby's bright blue eyes scan passing cars, bustling trucks and mammoth billboards. His gaze fixes on a motorist waiting for the traffic signal to turn green. I am the motorist.

"What am I doing here?" the baby's insistent eyes ask.

"Good question," I reply.

The light remains red.

"Well?" he persists.

"Don't know," I shrug.

A green light frees me from the infant's unanswerable question.

Just auditioned for one of the many Silicon Valley giants taking over Planet Earth. As I hurtle towards my next appointment, I scan the AM dial for companionship.

"If one of the parents can't be home all the time," says an accusatory, female voice, "they've got no business having children."

"But, what if my husband and I both have to work?" pleads a desperate caller.

"You should have thought about that before you got pregnant."

Francesca's company is moving to the other side of town, forty-five minutes away from our home. When she returns to work after maternity leave, she'll leave early in the morning and return well after dark.

"I can't be a full-time dad. I'll go crazy," I tell myself. "My career will come to a crashing halt. I'll end up doing what women have been forced to do for hundreds of generations."

I am in awe of my mother. I am in awe of all mothers. I am overwhelmed by their sacrifice.

I find myself thinking about a nanny, an eight-hour-a-day, in-house nanny. I never thought I'd consider a full-time nanny. I've spent a lifetime mocking the nanny-people.

My thoughts remind me of a conversation with Victor, an ex-Air Force pilot. One day we found ourselves, as always, involved in an intense discussion about my contemporaries. Out of the blue, Victor said, "I feel sorry for your generation."

"Huh?" I asked in disbelief. "Our generation is much better off than yours. We've got the Internet. We've got ATMs. We've got PlayStations."

"You can never be happy," he said, ignoring my sarcasm. "You expect to have everything. There's no concept of sacrifice. The idea of struggling is unacceptable. You expect to have perfect kids, keep your vacations, drive fancy cars, and spend money like there's no tomorrow. And, if one of those elements is missing, you feel put upon and dissatisfied."

"That's not true," I protested. "Maybe, ninety percent true. But not one hundred percent true."

Victor smiled knowingly.

"Okay," I relented, "so it's one hundred percent true."

I know many people who delayed parenthood until they amassed enough money to have it all. I know people who spent themselves into debt just to keep their lifestyles afloat after their baby arrived.

A lumbering garbage truck cuts in front of me.

When I got married, its magnitude overwhelmed me. In front of my family and my closest friends, I pledged to love and cherish Francesca 'til death do us part. The stakes seemed so high. Today a wedding looks like a walk in the park. Nice people feeding squirrels. Hot dog vendors offering fresh, steaming frankfurters. Soft pretzels at your beck and call. Friendly ducks quacking happily. Becoming a dad seems like a walk in a different kind of park. An abandoned park. In a bad neighborhood. At night. In the winter.

I speed past yet another Starbucks.

Throughout my life I have faced many crossroads. Each offered the opportunity to resist or embrace a new challenge. Every time I accepted the unknown I was better for the wear. When I resisted, I found myself unhappy and unfulfilled. Becoming a father is my next crossroad, another chance to travel an uncharted course. Staying in one place stunts the soul. Lingering lulls spirit into decay. I relish the approaching unknown.

Friday evening. Francesca emerges from an office building's darkly tinted front doors. Her shoulders sag underneath the weight of a laptop, handbag and wad of file folders. She struggles to climb inside our tiny Miata. Her many belongings make the task almost impossible.

"I'm so tired," Francesca says. Her distraught, empty eyes remind me of a marathoner who has just realized there are still ten miles to go.

A sudden, inexplicable surge of energy overrides the profound weariness. "Let's go out!" she declares gleefully.

"Sounds great," I say, yielding to the logic of hormones and pregnancy madness.

Francesca secures her seatbelt. "We're going to Burbank!"

"Burbank?" I embrace the madness. "Burbank it is."

"Perry?"

I've missed the Burbank exit. Perhaps Francesca's state is contagious.

"How about Pasadena?" I say without missing a beat.

"Pasadena? Sounds great."

Something tells me if I'd just said, "How about Las Vegas?" Francesca would have said "Las Vegas? Sounds great."

Miraculously we find a parking space in Pasadena's desirable Old Town shopping district. I fill the hungry parking meter with an endless stream of quarters.

"I love this place!" Francesca hops out of the car and bolts into a kitchen store.

Every food preparation device imaginable surrounds us: pasta makers, bread machines, and waffle irons. You name a food, and there's a machine here to puree it.

Francesca zeroes in on a saleswoman "Do you have slicing discs for the DL-10 Cuisinart?"

"We do," says the woman proudly. "It's one hundred and twenty five dollars."

"I'll take it."

"Take what?" I inquire. "What did we just take?"

Francesca grabs her shopping bag and darts across the street to a French Connection clothing store. A grating, monotonous beat blasts from an armada of deceptively small Bose speakers. One decibel more and my ears will bleed.

"I've been looking for these forever." Francesca grabs eight pairs of black socks and carries them to the front counter.

"Thirty-four dollars," reports the shell-shocked cashier.

"For socks?" I ask myself.

"Look," exclaims Francesca. "J. Crew!"

I scamper across a busy boulevard, hoping to keep up with my wife. I wonder if we'll max the Visa card before dinner.

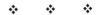

"My breasts hurt. I'm so tired. Honey, I'm so tired. Is this normal? Am I supposed to feel so tired? I've never felt this way. I feel so guilty for doing nothing and just being tired. So sleepy. So tired. My breasts hurt. My back hurts. My stomach feels twisted. I'm so sleeeee…"

Francesca falls into a deep, dense sleep.

Our six-cylinder, four-door sedan roars to life. I feel wildly rebellious in this automobile. I grew up in a Volkswagen family. My parents drove a gray Squareback and an orange Rabbit. Sitting behind the wheel of a car with automatic transmission, power door locks and poor gas mileage feels downright blasphemous. It makes me believe I've finally atoned for my overly obedient teenage years.

Francesca's random location selector, the one that delivered us to Pasadena last week, is now sending us to the science museum and its Imax theater.

We choose two center seats and sit down before a massive, four-story movie screen. "Everest," announces the ten-foot tall title credits. Spectacular, terrifying images flash one after the other. A Portuguese climber carefully crosses a deep crevasse, gingerly walking on an outstretched aluminum ladder. A freak blizzard claims the lives of mountaineers high up on the summit. A Sherpa weeps as he places his deceased father's photo at the top of the world.

The film ends in a blink. I help Francesca out of her chair and ponder the physicality of the climbers' quest. Sheer cliffs and loose rocks demanded the climbers' complete attention. None had time to obsess about quarterly taxes, bank balances, credit card debt, and future childcare. They thought only of their next steps. The climb freed them from the madness of everyday life. A thought occurs to me: Maybe I'd be happier if I started living more physically instead of playing host to my ever-obsessing mind. Perhaps jogging, bike riding, or digging holes in the backyard would bring more pleasure than worrying about financing my baby's education. Maybe I should approach the world as a champion climber, looking no further than my next step, propelled by simple, clear goals. Perhaps I should become an Urban Sherpa, a Mount Everest Dad. Another thought arrives with even greater profundity: I've lost my mind.

"What are you thinking about, sweetie?" asks Francesca.

"Nothing." Smart answer.

A pregnancy exhibit describes the various stages of gestation. Assorted diagrams and scale models illustrate the process.

"Week 8," states a stainless steel placard. "The organs are now distinct."

Our child could already have distinct organs. Parenthood rushes towards us. We examine the entire display. Francesca panics about how large her stomach will grow. I panic about everything. The Mount Everest euphoria vanishes.

Children explore fish tanks, microscopes and computer programs in a nearby exhibit hall.

"I can't wait to bring our baby here," I say aloud.

Francesca rubs her abdomen. "Neither can I."

Against our better judgment, we find ourselves at a bowling party.

Against our better judgment, we find ourselves having fun.

We meet an interesting couple, Richard and Evelyn. Richard and I hit it off immediately.

"Do you have children?" he asks.

"We'd like to. At some point. Not yet," I say, sticking to the party line.

"What do you do?"

"I'm an actor."

"Really?" his eyes light up.

"Yeah."

"I used to be an actor," he reflects.

"Really?"

"Until Sophie was born. Then I had to start making real money. Do you know how expensive childcare is?"

I drown my sorrows in a pitcher of Diet Coke.

Sunday greets us with blue skies and a light breeze. We coast down a large boulevard without a care in the world. Francesca starts to cry.

"This is really hard." Tears stream down her cheeks. "I've never been so tired in my life. I feel defective."

"You're pregnant, honey."

"I love you." Her eyes look deeply into mine. "How'd I ever find you?" Just as quickly, her eyes harden. Arms cross. "I want to have the baby now. I want my body back. I'm sick of being pregnant."

"Uh-huh," I say.

Her face brightens. A smile creeps across her mouth. "Maybe I'm not pregnant. We haven't had the sonogram yet."

"I think it's safe to say you're pregnant."

Darkness again. "I feel nauseous. I'm sick."

"We'll be home soon. Here, drink some water." I hand her a large bottle of Evian. "You'll feel better."

Francesca's eyes well up. Her face beams at me and then collapses into tears. "You're the nicest man I've ever known."

"Honey—"

"—No I mean it. You're so wonderful and cute and lovable."

I hand her a box of Kleenex.

"Look, you gave me Kleenex without my having to ask. You're so thoughtful. I love you."

"I love you, too."

A torrent of new tears flow forth.

"I guess I'm a little emotional right now."

Francesca models a cute green blouse.

"It looks good, honey, but it doesn't offer much room to grow."

Francesca disappears behind a dressing room curtain. A minute later, she emerges, her face filled with rage.

"I must have said something that hurt your feelings," I say, illustrating my unique ability to state the obvious.

My wife replies with silence, a turn of the back and an angry march out the front door. I trail behind, weaving my way through pierced pedestrians.

"Was it the 'It doesn't offer much room to grow' comment?" I inquire as if I don't already know the answer is "Yes."

"I don't want to talk about it here," snaps Francesca. She bounds across the street, dodging passing cars, motorcycles and buses.

I chase after my wife, trying to close the gap between us.

"Please tell me what's wrong," I call to her.

"You can never do anything just for fun. Everything has to be practical. For a reason."

"Huh?"

"I'm not fat yet, okay? I can buy a blouse for right now if I want," Francesca's voice rises to a roar.

"Sure you can," I say, sensing impending doom.

"Not with you." Her claws extend. "You control everything. I pay for the mortgage. But I'm not allowed to spend a dime on clothes."

"That's not true."

"Yes it is! You're always controlling me. Telling me what to do. This is such bullshit."

She circles the prey.

"You want that blouse?" I yell. "Let's go back and get the blouse. I thought you were looking for pregnancy clothes."

"Did I say I was looking for pregnancy clothes?" screams Francesca. "Did I?"

I think about the question for a moment. "I thought you did."

"Well, I didn't. Maybe if you learned to listen, you'd know how I really feel. Who knows? Maybe the baby's dead. Maybe I'm not pregnant."

The kill.

"Francesca, don't say that."

"See, there you go again, controlling me. I want to leave. Now."

We drive home without speaking a word. Francesca turns away from me and stares at passing storefronts.

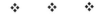

Francesca opens a window and watches me mow the lawn. I know exactly what she's thinking.

"You want a blow job?" she asks, the exact opposite of what I knew she was thinking.

I stop mowing. The grass can wait.

"How'd it go?" I ask.

"Il ooo di poo."

A cacophony of distorted noises overwhelms Francesca's answer.

"Huh?"

"Zlee they meen and cass."

I strain to separate Francesca's words from odd electronic thuds and squeals, the unmistakable trademarks of crystal-clear, digital cell phone technology.

"It didn't!" She sounds like the Terminator.

"What happened?"

"They couldn't administer the bloozen."

"Honey?" Snap. "I missed that last part." Crackle. "Honey?" Pop.

"Can you hear me?" she shouts through the binary blizzard.

"Now I can," I yell. "What happened?"

"They wouldn't give me the sonogram because they need some special referral form from Doctor Braintree."

"So what happens now?" I speak rapidly, hoping to finish the call before the next, inevitable hi-tech glitch.

"What?" Francesca's voice sounds tinny, as if we're communicating with empty frozen orange juice cans connected by string.

"So what happens now?" I ask again.

"Can you hear me now?" Her voiceprint returns to its familiar pattern.

"What happens now?"

"I have to wait until Doctor Braintree returns from his leave."

"That's a month away."

"I know."

"We can't wait that long."

"Perry, I can't deal with this bullshit right wooo!"

"What?"

"It doesn't hooblit. Blee are early in the pregnoon any geewan."

"Do you want me to talk to them?" I offer.

"No. I can oseal of it," she says firmly. "I muntee."

"Francesca? Hello? Hello?"

Elevator doors open wide to a sweeping view of our health center's main lobby. Strangers thrust together by illness concoct unsuccessful strategies to endure hour-long delays.

"Can I help you?" inquires a haggard receptionist. Claim forms cover every inch of her semicircular desk.

"My wife just had a terrible experience here. I want to speak with whoever runs this office." My eyes are firm, but kind.

"One moment." She disappears behind a doorway.

"Mr. Herman?" A thirty-something, tastefully dressed woman leads me to her office. "I'm Mrs. Wright," she says, offering a chair.

"Nice to meet you."

"What seems to be the matter?" she asks mechanically.

"My wife was just denied a sonogram because she doesn't have a referral form from her doctor."

"That's the policy," continues the drone. "Your insurance company requires referral forms for all services."

A strained smile vanishes from my face. "See, I know that, only we can't get a referral form from our doctor. He's on leave."

"That's a problem." The administrator hunches over her desk. Her shoulders droop under the weight of a gargantuan corporate bureaucracy, which, according to today's new-economy gurus, is somehow preferable to gargantuan government bureaucracy.

"Francesca is more than two months pregnant." My cheeks travel clockwise through the color wheel from light pink to red.

"She's too busy to show up for an exam and be denied care. So here's what's going to happen. You will find three available appointment times for tomorrow. You will then call Francesca and ask her which is most convenient. Got it?"

"Got it," responds the administrator. "If you ask me," she continues, suddenly inspired by my militancy, "The policy stinks."

For a split second we revel in our mini-uprising, galvanized by visions of the Boston Tea Party and Norma Rae.

A piercing rendition of *Yankee Doodle Dandy* erupts from my ocean blue Ericsson.

"This is Perry."

"What did you do?" demands Francesca.

"Why?"

"Someone just called from the clinic offering me three appointment times."

"I took care of business."

The quiet hiss of a vacant phone line is my only reply.

"Honey?" I inquire.

"No one's ever done that for me." Francesca's voice quivers.

"Made an appointment?"

"No. Taken care of something for me. Like that. Thank you."

"Francesca, I love you. This is what you do when you love someone."

"It's just," her voice becomes unstable. "Everything is so crazy. Work's completely insane. I'm tired. I feel nauseous and, half the time, I can't even remember my name. I love you."

"I love you, too."

"You're a good man, Perry Herman."

No one has ever said that to me before. The feeling is indescribable. I feel full. I feel buoyant. I feel honorable.

As my car crawls through bumper-to-bumper traffic, I feel a sense of relief, thrilled I didn't miss a key moment, the first images of our baby. Francesca had been so insistent: "I'll go alone. It's no big deal." Everything is a big deal. I vow never to skip a doctor visit.

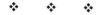

The first blood tests are back. Everything reads normal. So far, so good.

My pager vibrates. An unfamiliar phone number materializes on its liquid crystal display.

"Hello?" I ask cautiously, uncertain of my audience. A drug dealer could have inadvertently dialed my pager. A kidnapper could have mistakenly beeped me. If I am responding to a criminal's misguided page, I pray he doesn't have *69 service.

"Where are you?" It's not a drug dealer or a kidnapper. It's my wife.

"Where am I? I'm on my way to the sonogram."

"It just happened."

"What just happened?"

"The sonogram."

"The appointment wasn't until one o'clock."

"I had to move it up. There's a crisis at work."

Disappointment floods my body. I've just missed the first view of our fetus. I've missed it.

"Wanna grab some food?" Francesca's unexpected offer softens the blow. We never lunch together on weekdays. Her endless stream of business appointments makes it impossible. "Woo Fat," she declares. "Twenty minutes."

I scan a sea of restaurant patrons and, in a far corner, locate Francesca's beaming face. I've never seen her radiate this way. Her smile is infectious. She grins. I grin.

We order mixed vegetable tofu, vegetable pot stickers and beef with broccoli.

"I'm nine weeks pregnant," she says.

"How does everything look?"

"Everything looks good."

Dumplings miraculously arrive at our table.

"How about Roma Gabrielle Manarola Herman?" Francesca gobbles a glistening chicken dumpling.

"For what?"

"If it's a girl."

"I love the name Roma, you know that."

"How about Giovanni Hugo Giuseppe Vincenzo Manarola?"

"If it's a boy?"

"Yes!" cheers Francesca.

"It doesn't sound too Jewish." My ancestors gasp in horror. "What happened to Max?"

Tofu with vegetables.

Beef with broccoli.

Two iced teas.

Three glasses of water.

Two trips to the restroom.

The check.

The yellow credit card receipt.

A kiss.

Another kiss.

A goodbye.

The red Miata pulls away from the curb, accelerates down the street and stops suddenly. Francesca sticks her head out the window and beckons me to say goodbye once more. I lean into the car and kiss her.

"You're going to be a great mom," I say.

"You're going to be a great dad," she says.

Francesca nibbles on a cracker. "I can't even think straight, Perry. I feel exhausted. My stomach's twisting."

I know Francesca wants me to say, "You should stay home." Her devout work ethic forbids her from taking a sick day.

"You should stay home," I say.

"Really?" Her eyes brighten.

"Yes," I continue. "Call in sick. Normal people call in sick all the time."

"Really?" She tests me once again.

"Really."

"I'm sick," she proclaims.

"Yes, you are."

"I'm not going to work. I'm sick."

"Yes."

Francesca slumps under the bed sheets. "Can I have some ginger ale?"

"You can have whatever you want."

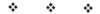

"And as you lay on this magic carpet, you make a second wish, a wish for something you may not have yet." The calming tones of my acting coach float through the rehearsal studio. I am in the midst of a sensory exercise, a physical exploration of imaginary objects and spaces. My classmates and I reach through the air and gradually "discover" our wishes. If an unsuspecting person walked into the studio right now, he'd assume he'd stumbled upon a psychiatric ward.

When I work well in a sensory exercise, the experience is fully spontaneous. My body physically leads me to unknown places and things. Tonight I am working well. I find myself holding something. My fingers explore its surface. I discover a soft texture, one that suggests skin. My forearm senses an object spanning a foot, a distance from my hand to my elbow. It moves. Fingers. Legs. A nose. I'm holding my baby.

I feel embarrassed in front of the other students. It makes no sense, since everyone else looks equally ridiculous holding their imaginary objects. I force myself to go deeper into the exploration. I move to the floor and "play" with my baby. Its legs twirl. Its arms flail.

"Now, let that object go. You're third wish is next."

I ignore my coach and stay with my second wish. It's too good to leave. Fatherhood. Coming soon to a theater near you.

Nick, Francesca's brother, hacks away at a hole in the backyard. I shovel dirt out of a small ditch. We are planting two Brisbane Box trees in the hope that—some day—these fledgling plants will obscure our next door neighbor's towering house.

"Lunch!" Francesca bursts from the kitchen carrying a plate full of sandwiches.

We sit around the plastic patio table, our faces barely shielded from the sun by a woefully small umbrella. The rising heat bakes us unmercifully as we devour peanut butter and jelly sandwiches.

"Do my breasts look bigger?" Francesca asks her brother.

"Well…" he begins.

I stare into Nick's eyes and discretely shake my head "No."

"No," he answers. "They look the same."

"Do I seem bigger to you?" she persists.

Once again, my head shakes no.

"Not at all," says Nick, too forcefully. "In fact, you look skinnier." He looks to me for approval. I offer him a discrete "thumbs up," even though his credibility just went down the tubes.

"Perry?" Francesca moves to me for a more reliable, second opinion.

"Nope," I say assuredly. "No change as far as I can see."

She is not convinced. We finish lunch and return to our holes.

Francesca breezes into the house just as the hour hand passes six o'clock. Thirty years ago people regularly returned home at six. This isn't thirty years ago. This is the Internet Age, the "I'll be home at midnight" era. I wonder if something is wrong.

Francesca prances into the kitchen. "I'm going to bake you a pie!"

Pots, pans and baking sheets clank loudly. Glass jars and cooking utensils clatter on tile counter tops. I sneak into the foyer and fish through Francesca's handbag looking for a pink slip or new medication.

"Do you want a peach or apricot pie?" she yells from the pantry.

"Apricot," I reply, still suspicious of my audience.

"I'm going to bake my husband a pie."

An extensive search of Francesca's black, Kate Spade bag reveals no incriminating evidence. No pink slip. No medication. No arrest warrants. All I uncover is a half-opened pack of Trident, which, unless I'm mistaken, cannot explain her strange behavior.

"I think I'll make some shortbread, too."

Who bakes shortbread, I ask myself? "Can't wait!" I say aloud.

"Where's that fabulous Martha Stewart recipe?"

I peer into the kitchen. Francesca ricochets between rolling dough, mixing flour and slicing fruit.

"I'm going to make the best apricot pie ever!" she exclaims.

"That's great, honey."

I'm checking the handbag again.

"I watered all the plants!" Francesca awakens me from a horrible sleep. An armada of police helicopters, birds, barking dogs and an angry woodpecker kept me up all last night.

"Good…yes…good," I sputter.

"I did some dishes, and I'll be heading out the door soon." Francesca plants a warm kiss on my cheek.

"Good…yes…good." I try to remember my name.

A slow, leftward body roll places my face squarely in front of our clock radio. "5:53," it shines.

"The trees are so happy." Francesca rifles through her closet, evaluating potential outfits for the day.

"5:53," I mumble.

"Oh…it's early."

"Uh-huh."

"I guess the baby woke me up."

"I guess so."

Dark, bloodshot eyes stare back at me from the medicine cabinet mirror. My bright orange Reach toothbrush falls from my mouth. In an exuberant flourish, Francesca finishes her make-up. Even in my exhausted haze, I can still appreciate her strong eyebrows and full lips.

"I love you," she whispers in my ear.

The front door closes.

The front door opens.

A groan. A sigh.

Francesca limps past me. She clutches her stomach and collapses on our bed.

"Saltines and sparkling water, coming up." I say, already halfway to the kitchen.

Francesca drinks water and nibbles a cracker. Her demeanor improves. She stands upright, smiles and, once again, bravely marches out the door.

Metallica bleeds from outdoor speakers. Scantily clad partygoers thrash about in a pool. A woman parading in a high cut, one-piece bathing suit bears an uncanny resemblance to the ideal Playboy playmate. I try not to stare as I pour my pregnant wife a glass of tonic water.

"I'm so sick of sparkling water," Francesca bemoans. "Lemon sparkling water. Lime sparkling water. Lemon-lime sparkling water."

A crowd of people surrounds a giant Bud Light keg. Golden beer flows continuously from the tap. A man licks foam off his index finger.

"Go ahead," Francesca says. "Have one. Tell me what it's like."

"Are you sure?"

"Perry," she says with an edge, "you're not pregnant."

The amber liquid flows smoothly down my throat.

"How is it?"

"It's okay," I lie.

"You're lying."

"It's fantastic," I confess.

A young couple clutching identical babies walks past us. The father artfully feeds one of the infants with a tiny milk bottle.

"Wow. Twins," spills from my mouth.

"Wow is right!" says the father. "It's been nonstop since they were born." Despite his wearied state, he wears a gleeful smile.

"How old?" inquires Francesca.

"Four months." The new mom wraps a baby in a warm, pink blanket.

"What's it like?" I ask a bit too eagerly.

"An unpaid, fulltime job," says the father.

There's a great second career for an actor, I think to myself. A day job that pays nothing.

"We tried to go it alone—without a nanny," laughs the father. "That lasted a week."

"What do you pay for child care?" I ask abruptly, not appreciating the humor.

"Two hundred fifty dollars a week."

A sudden, uncontrollable impulse compels me to concoct and solve a series of calculations:

$250 x 4 weeks = $1,000 per month
$1,000 x 12 months = $12,000 per year
$12,000 net = $20,000 gross

Panic courses through my veins.

"You expecting?" asks the father.

"Us? Oh no. Just asking. We want to have kids. But, no luck yet, you know."

He smiles knowingly. He recognizes the "pregnant-in-secret" dance.

"Well, I'll tell you something." He places his hand on my right shoulder. "It's the best, most incredible thing in the world—being a dad."

"Yeah?"

"I want to have more," he adds.

I finish my Bud Light.

"I'm so happy to see you again." Doctor Braintree embraces Francesca.

The teddy bear nurse smiles warmly. "Welcome back."

We stare at the tiny sonogram monitor, our eyes fixed on the familiar black and white wedge of apple pie. Francesca's body grows rigid in anticipation of the exam and its unknown results. I stroke her long brown hair, grit my teeth, and survey the mysterious data populating the right hand side of the screen: *12W20. 73cm. +02.*

"Ouch!" barks Francesca.

"What?"

"You're pulling my hair!"

"There's the fetus," our doctor reports as he moves the sonogram probe around Francesca's abdomen. The fetus' outline fills more of the screen than the first one ever did. "That's the femur." A solid diagonal line along the bottom edge of the pie slice. "There are the arms and the legs." Tiny mitten hands appear in the center of the screen. A head and the beginnings of a spine follow.

"The placenta is positioned low in the uterus," says Doctor Braintree. "The edge of it is overlapping the cervix."

"Placenta Previa?" asks Francesca.

"Could be, but we're still very early in the process. In many cases the placenta moves up the wall of the uterus and eventually reaches a normal position. I would recommend you refrain from intercourse for the time being."

"No intercourse?" I ask.

"None," he replies firmly.

"Perry, do you know what Placenta Previa is?"

"Huh?" I answer, uncertain of the connection between Placentia Previa and the stack of *People* magazines we're reading.

"During the exam yesterday," she continues, "the doctor noticed symptoms of Placenta Previa."

"Uh-huh." I look up at Francesca only to find myself face to face with a smiling Tom Hanks, *Hollywood's Favorite Star*.

"Didn't you hear him?"

"Well, yeah." I catch myself rereading the same movie review a third time.

Francesca disappears down the hallway and returns with a thick, hardbound reference book. Large uppercase letters overwhelm its dust cover: *THE MERCK MANUAL OF MEDICAL INFORMATION*. She opens the tome to an already bookmarked page.

"Normally, the placenta is located in the upper part of the uterus," she reads. My wife, the daughter of a doctor, speaks as if she's discussing one of her patient's symptoms. "The placenta may cover the opening of the cervix completely or partially." She skips a few lines and then rolls onward. "Painless vaginal bleeding begins suddenly in late pregnancy. When bleeding is profuse, repeated blood transfusions may be needed. When bleeding is minor and delivery isn't imminent, bed rest is usually advised. A cesarean section is almost always performed, because if the woman goes into labor, the placenta tends to become detached, depriving the baby of its oxygen supply. In addition, there may be massive bleeding in the mother."

Francesca shuts the book. Dark clouds swirl around her furrowed brow. For a moment I am speechless.

"Wait," I recover, "didn't he say the placenta often travels up the uterus into the right position?"

"Yes, but sometimes it doesn't," snaps Francesca.

"And a lot of times it does," I fire back, remembering that my wife is not, in fact, a trained physician. "This is going to be a healthy pregnancy."

The clouds break. A hint of sunlight shines through.

"What if it isn't?" persists Francesca.

I realize Francesca is gripped by fear. I realize she has been worrying about Placenta Previa since the exam.

"We were meant to be parents," I say resolutely.

"You really think so?" Francesca reaches for another dose of reassurance.

"I know so."

Francesca discards the *Merck Manual* in favor of *Star Tracks.*

"I don't want anything to go wrong this time," she whispers.

Our hands entwine. We hold one another. Her breathing slows.

"Let us have a healthy baby," I plead to no one in particular.

The universe offers no reply.

Coarse rain batters the plane's delicate hull. Lightning illuminates the straining propeller, visible through my tiny window. The twin engine island hopper lurches left, then right. Other passengers holler in fear. My hands grip slender, stainless steel hand rests. A thunder crack. A thud. A silence. The plane hesitates for a moment before it gracefully points its nose downward and begins a quiet plunge towards the tropical, tree covered land below. My mind empties itself of all thoughts. I am conscious of my breath. I prepare for the end.

Toxic fumes waft past me as my eyes open slowly. Flames leap about twisted remains of chairs, fuselage and bodies. Sharp pains shoot through my lower back, indicating I have somehow survived. A perilous crawl through jagged metal and shattered glass leads me to safety, a patch of smooth dirt. I moan and collapse into sleep.

I awaken again. My body rests on a rickety, makeshift staircase that leads to a flimsy, wooden hut. A tall, razor wire fence surrounds the entire structure. An unmistakable sound reverberates through the compound—the metallic click of a bullet locking into a rifle chamber. I run for the fence and find a small hole in the metal lattice. I struggle to pass through the twisted wire but my girth makes escape impossible. Fatigue closes in…

Coarse rain batters the plane's delicate hull. Lightning illuminates the straining propeller, visible through my tiny window. The twin engine island hopper lurches left, then right. Other passengers holler in fear. My hands grip slender, stainless steel hand rests. I'm back on the plane again. I have to live this again.

"Perry?" A stewardess calls out to me. I look up and down the center aisle.

"Perry?" The aisle fades into a fog.

"Perry!" I am in a hotel room.

"Perry!" Francesca calls to me.

"Francesca?"

"Are you alright?" she asks.

"Why?" My heart races.

"You were lying on your side and you were…running."

"Running?" Sweat beads from my forehead.

"You were running in place…on your side."

"I was the only survivor of a horrible plane crash. I was trapped in an island prison compound. There was no escape. No way out. I couldn't get through the fence. Then the whole thing started all over again."

Francesca takes me in her arms.

"It was horrible." My body relaxes in her embrace. "What do you think it was about?"

"Fatherhood," she answers without missing a beat.

"Fatherhood?"

"The plane crash is about leaving a world that is familiar to you—a world without children. And the prison is parenthood, a place from which there's no escape. Your dream repeats, meaning you'll have to live in this new place for the rest of your life."

I brace myself for two more trimesters of expectant dreams.

Magritte canvases encircle us.

Ceci n'est pas une pipe.

Ceci n'est pas un Magritte—Max Ernst.

We stand at the top level of New York's spiraling Guggenheim Museum. Paintings pass by us as we embark on a slow, downward descent. I peer over the precariously low railing and watch people dart back and forth on the ground floor below. Francesca pauses. She fights valiantly against worn muscles and aching feet.

"There's a great bench on the other side of that archway," I offer.

Francesca lies down on the long seat and rests her head on my lap. I caress her face—the thick eyebrows, the delicate nose, the beautiful mouth. Jaw muscles relax. Hands grow limp. Sleep comes.

Hundred-degree heat bakes us and the other unfortunate pedestrians traversing Madison Avenue. We duck into a Crate and Barrel in search of air conditioning and a gift for my brother's wife. The utensil section contains the perfect present, an innovative wine bottle corker. A cashier wraps the gift delicately and places it inside a crisp, white shopping bag. We linger in the store, basking in super-cooled air while we build the courage to leave. A final sigh propels us out the door and back into the oppressively humid air. Our legs carry us past a hot dog vendor and a barking French poodle. My back grows damp. Shirtsleeves stick to my skin.

Francesca makes an abrupt left turn. I trail behind her, trying to imagine what has suddenly captured her attention. A snaking corridor leads us to a store filled with racks and racks of clothes. Mimi Maternity heralds a large banner hanging from the ceiling. Francesca disappears into a changing room and emerges in a red, daisy-print sundress.

"What do you think?" she asks nervously.

"What do I think?"

"You hate it!"

"No."

"Well?"

"It's just that…" I try to find the words.

"What?" she stomps towards the dressing area. "I'll take it off."

"You look so cute."

Francesca stops. "Really?"

"Yes." The knee-length dress cascades over her pale white legs. Its red hue warms her already glowing cheeks.

"Should I buy it?"

"Absolutely."

I want her to wear this dress for the next five months.

The first act of "Rent" catapults us into an excited reverie. We join a throng of theatergoers milling about on the street just outside the auditorium. A smartly dressed man feverishly inhales a cigarette while his date checks voicemail. An improvisational dance troop assembles just beyond the curb and churns to the percussion of a garbage can drummer. Angry cabbies protest the clogged street with repeated honks and curses.

An aging, African American man appears before us, his eyes bloodshot. "I'm not begging. I'm selling a newspaper about the homeless. It's a way for—" The pitch halts abruptly. "It's gonna be a girl," he says assuredly.

"What?" The unsolicited prediction startles Francesca.

"Your baby is going to be a girl."

"How do you know?"

"I've had twelve kids myself. Believe me, I know." He pauses for a moment, then rubs his chin. "How many months pregnant are you?"

"Guess," asks the intrigued mother-to-be.

"Almost five months."

"Four and a half," she confirms.

"See?" The old man chuckles to himself. "What did I tell you?"

I purchase a newspaper. "Keep the change," I tell our soothsayer.

The oracle smiles, waves *The Homeless Times* in the air, and approaches his next customer.

"I guess we're having a girl," I say.

"Who needs a sonogram?" remarks Francesca.

The house lights flicker on and off. Arms intertwined, we return to the lavish lobby and prepare for the second act.

Gate seventy-three, John F. Kennedy Airport. A week in New York ends all too soon. Regular, day-to-day concerns sneak back into my thoughts—bills, overdue letters, meetings, opportunities, unknowns.

"Move!" snaps Francesca.

"Huh?"

"We don't know each other."

"Huh?"

"People from work just showed up."

We hide behind a stainless steel column.

"She's in marketing. He's in sales." A man wrapped in dark sunglasses and an Armani suit approaches us. An equally fashionable woman follows close behind.

None of Francesca's coworkers know I joined her in New York. It's not that we've done anything wrong. Spouses often accompany executives during extended business trips. *Wives*, that is, regularly travel with their husbands.

Female department heads, unlike their male counterparts, must always appear independent and *available* in the work world. Women must not only sell their intelligence, ingenuity and total commitment to work, but also their sexuality. I understand the situation.

"You board the plane first," she lays out the battle plan. "I'll get on five minutes later and, when I sit down next to you, we won't know each other."

Francesca disappears into a crowd. Her flower-print dress, new shoes and Mimi Maternity shopping bag vanish behind bodies and carry-on luggage. My eyes widen in horror. Mimi Maternity. I can feel the absolute danger of the moment. I assume the role of an agent on deep cover, circle around the lobby, and then head straight for Francesca. She glares at me with wide, disparaging eyes: *You're not following the plan.*

"Excuse me," I say, as if a stranger.

"What are you doing?" she growls under her breath.

"The bag," I whisper.

"What about it?"

"Look what's printed on it!"

A moment of horror. "Oh my God," she gasps.

"Drop it. Take my bag."

"You're good. You're really good." Francesca grabs my bag. I grab hers. I walk away. Mission accomplished.

I find my seat, peer out the window and admire a view of metal rivets, wing flaps and the phrase *No Step.* I page through the in-flight magazine, anxious to discover the movie I'll be forced to watch. I think of all the films that tanked in the last four months, knowing one will be the *Premier Presentation.* I find the entertainment listings. Bingo. *It's spring break again in this feel-good, coming-of-age comedy starring today's brightest young stars.*

"Excuse me sir, is this your bag?" Francesca asks, pointing at our yellow backpack.

"Oh, yes. I'm sorry. I'll stow it."

"Thank you."

Francesca sits next to me, grabs a pen and scribbles furiously on the back of an airsickness bag.

"The marketing director is sitting right behind you," she writes.

"I guess that rules out handholding," I write back.

"Yes," she confirms.

Our correspondence moves to another vomit bag.

"Does this mean we can't talk?" I continue.

"Yes."

"Why can't you happen to strike up a conversation with me? We'll just be two strangers on a plane talking."

"I don't want to attract any attention."

"What if we were on separate business trips and just happened to be taking the same flight home?"

"Too coincidental."

"I love you, even though you're a total stranger."

Francesca composes a tic-tac-toe grid, places the first X and motions me to make my first move.

"My name is Perry." I write instead.

Francesca grimaces.

"You are so beautiful," I say in cursive letters. "Will you marry me and have my baby?"

Francesca skips my turn and places another X.

The movie lasts forever. It's unbearable, even without the sound. I finish a small brick of "gourmet" lasagna and wolf down a tasteless garden salad. Mind numbing commercials disguised as news magazines pollute the cabin for another three hours.

"Pardon me." Francesca grabs our bag, finds her balance and plods up the center aisle. The marketing director follows close behind. I remain seated, pretending to be entranced by a product in the *Sky Emporium* catalog, a poster featuring a bald eagle and the word *Strength*.

As I step off of the jet-way, I see Francesca talking with her coworkers. She mouths the words, baggage claim. I nod.

Miraculously, our luggage appears moments after the carousel starts. We leave the other passengers behind to determine which black roller bags are their black roller bags.

Francesca taps my shoulder. "We're clear."

"Positive?"

"Yes, we're clear."

I spin around and plant a kiss squarely on my wife's lips.

Nine-fifty in the morning. Francesca lies on an examination table. I sit forward in a cushioned, metal chair. We smile at each another. Our strained faces betray our anxiety.

"Has the placenta moved upwards?" Francesca ruminates silently.

"Can we have sex again?" I wonder.

Doctor Braintree enters the cramped room, carrying a small device.

"Where's the sonogram?" I blurt, blowing my cover as the calm, confident man.

"In the other room," he answers matter-of-factly. He wears a threadbare dress shirt and pants belted high above his midriff.

"Don't we need one?" I continue, as if I'm the one with the medical degree.

"Not today," he responds without a shred of disgust. Thirty years of experience must make a physician immune to second-guessing, expectant fathers.

The doctor rubs Francesca's stomach with a clear gel, activates the small device and slides it around the abdominal area.

"Wooozee-Ahhhhh!" The sound of a screaming alien leaps from the appliance. It screams again and again, more urgently with each cry. "Zeee-Bap! Zee-Wap!" A sudden succession of fast *pings* follow: Ping! Ping! Ping! Ping! Ping! The alien cry of mercy returns. "Wooozee-Bum!" Another ping. Another yelp. A ping. A scream. A ping. A screech.

"That's the baby moving," reports the doctor. "—And that..." Ping. Ping. Ping. Ping. "...is its heartbeat."

I beam. Our baby. Its heart beating.

We've reached the fourth month mark. The odds improve.

Francesca peers out a small, airtight window. She contemplates the wing tip and its flashing crimson light. We are traveling to San Francisco for a wedding shower. A grinning flight attendant named Anne offers us a microscopic bag of peanuts.

"Uuuh!" Francesca clutches her stomach.

"What? What is it?" I prepare for the worst. An emergency landing. CPR in the aisle.

"Enrico kicked me."

"He did?"

"He kicked me. Hard." Francesca grips her midsection. "There. There he goes again. Wham! Put your hand there." I put my hand there.

"Do you feel it?" she asks. "Do you?"

As much as I want to, I feel nothing.

"He stopped." Francesca's right hand grips my left. "He kicked, Perry, our son kicked!"

A moment. A pause.

"Who's Enrico?" I ask.

"That's our son's name."

"Our son?"

"Yes."

"It's a good name. I like it."

"Me, too."

"When did we decide on Enrico?"

"Just now."

"When did we know Enrico is a boy?"

"Just now."

"What about the prophet of New York?"

"It's a boy." Francesca chews on a peanut. "I know it."

A mattress and box spring lean against a hallway wall. Side tables, reading lamps and luggage populate the living room. Chaos.

Painters will soon descend upon our house to embark on *Phase Three* of construction. I've begun to wonder what we actually acquired when we bought our 1936 Spanish charmer. It's as if we took delivery on an automobile, only to discover it had no engine.

Francesca and I lay on the narrow guest bed in Enrico's room. Francesca clutches what is becoming her most prized possession: a pink, four-foot long, down feather pillow.

"He's up again," she announces. "Put your hand on my stomach."

I place my hand on Francesca's stomach.

"Push down."

I push down ever so lightly.

"Harder. You won't hurt him."

I push harder and feel a new firmness in Francesca's abdomen. It pushes back with as much strength as I can apply.

"Do you feel him?"

I feel nothing.

"Move your hand around the upper right side of my stomach."

I move my hand upward and to the right. My palm tingles. I sense something in my fingers.

"There he is!" My eyes open wide, staring into the darkness. "Right there." I pinpoint the location with my index finger. A succession of kicks and thumps follows.

"Wow!" is all I can think to say. "Wow!"

"He's never going to give me a rest," laments an exhausted Francesca.

I lean down and, for the first time, find myself talking to Enrico: "Hi, Enrico. It's Dad. Your mom is trying to sleep. You think you could stop kicking for a few seconds, just so she can relax a bit?"

I wait for a response.

"Ugh!" grunts Francesca.

It's Enrico's swiftest kick yet. A firm, determined thrust.

"Well, we know one thing," I observe.

"What's that?" asks Francesca.

"Our child has a definite point of view."

"I bought us another home!" Francesca announces with glee.

"Say again?"

"I bought us another home!"

"When? With what?"

"Come on! I want you to see it!"

Francesca grabs my hand, brings me outside and leads me up a steep incline. We stand at the front door of a rambling Mediterranean home. Its white plaster facade, lush front lawn and sweeping city views are stunning. Francesca produces a shiny brass key, smiles, unlocks the front door and leads me inside our new abode. Lush Mexican tile covers the floor. I walk around the foyer, climb a staircase and find myself in a second floor library. I gaze out of the windows and see the Hollywood sign clearly.

"We own this?" I ask.

"Yup!" her voice echoes from below.

One corner of the room seems unusually bright. I notice a warm pool of light illuminating the wooden flooring. I crane my head upward to find its source. The origin is clear as day—a gaping hole in the roof. I become aware of massive cracks in the walls throughout. The floor creaks strangely. I rush downstairs to alert Francesca. She is nowhere to be found. I run outside and discover the house is now rundown and abandoned.

"Currently it's seventy-five degrees downtown and sixty-nine degrees along the coast."

I open my eyes, looking for the source of the sound. I find it. My clock radio.

"Whatever happened to simple happy dreams with flowers and birds?" I wonder aloud.

"Huh?" mutters Francesca, her voice muffled by her giant, pink body pillow.

"I said, 'Good morning.'"

"Morning," she replies sleepily.

I consider the pink pillow. Inexplicably, its presence fills me with foreboding. Its unnatural proportions suggest something obscene and unsettling.

"Francesca?" I close the front door behind me. "Honey?" I move slowly through the house, not wanting to startle my wife.

"Over here," trickles down the hallway. I know the voice. The voice of surrender. The voice of defeat.

I follow Francesca's whisper into Enrico's bedroom. She lies on her back, her arms extended out above her head, her legs stretched apart. Her body forms a human X.

"I told Alan," she says. Alan. A co-worker at Francesca's company.

"And?"

"At first he said 'Five months pregnant? Why'd you keep it a secret?'" Francesca sits up, her eyes empty. "Then he said, 'Are you coming back?' And I said 'Coming back where?' He gave me this look and said, 'To work. You never know until you hold that baby.'" A deep sigh. "He'd never ask a man that question."

My wife has worked tirelessly for her company. She has made innumerable sacrifices to provide value, control costs and streamline production. She lives music. She breathes music. This is her career.

"I feel like a marked man," she laments. "Now that I'm pregnant, I'm out of the game. Thank God I waited as long as I did."

"He's acting as if you've got cancer," I observe.

"By the way," Francesca stares over the edge of the bed. "My company was just voted a top business for working mothers. It's celebrating by giving everyone Friday off."

I rub Francesca's forehead.

"It's so unfair." She curls into my chest and starts to cry.

❖ 4 ❖

We embrace in the Lufthansa lobby, a voluminous circular space punctuated by doorways leading to waiting airplanes. My stomach presses against Francesca's abdomen. A familiar sensation greets me—a succession of rhythmic taps. *Tap tap tap.* Enrico kicks left. *Tap tap tap.* Enrico kicks right.

With every passing day, Enrico becomes more of a reality, more of a presence in our lives. He is with us wherever we go. Francesca moves differently. Her feet flare out, transforming her walk into a waddle. Her swelling abdomen forces her spine into an inward curve. My attention wanders away from career. Francesca's balance, breathing, and emotions dominate my thoughts.

Nineteen hours separate us from Switzerland, our final destination. *Tap tap tap.* I wonder if Enrico is preparing for the flight.

Subzero temperatures envelop the airplane. We twist and turn in the inhumanely small Lufthansa coach seats. It dawns on me that today is Rosh Hashanah. I am traveling on a German jumbo jet on the highest Jewish holiday. Perhaps the uncomfortable chairs are not a fluke. Perhaps they are the first in a series of punishments meted out by my creator. The seat just ahead of me lunges backward, jamming my feet beneath its thinly cushioned back. God confirms my theory.

My eyes close. They open. I pray our journey's end is near. I glance at an overhead monitor. It displays a world map and the position of our plane: thirty-two thousand feet above Chicago.

"I have to get up." Francesca leads me to a tiny open space near an exit hatch, kneels, and then leans backward until her spine lies firmly on the floor.   A flight attendant regards us dismissively. *What do you coach people think you're doing?*

"My wife is pregnant," I spurt. "She's feeling nauseous."

The stewardess' face softens. "I've got just the trick!" She unfolds a jump seat and urges me to sit. She instructs Francesca to raise her feet and rest them on my lap. Francesca exhales in relief. New York slips beneath us.

My eyes close. They open. The television above reveals Iceland lies below. Francesca and I seek refuge in our headphones. Boy bands. Speed metal. Bavarian accordion music. No luck.

My eyes close. They open. Iceland refuses to budge. My mind whirs, locked in an infinite loop. The house, the finances, the baby, Francesca, and the alarm system. The house, the finances, the baby, Francesca, and the alarm system.

Geneva Airport. Francesca's cousin Frédérique greets her bleary-eyed relatives. Our bodies collapse into the back seat of a battered Toyota sedan. Streetlights and taxis whiz past us. An ambulance rumbles through an intersection, its siren wailing.

"C'est impossible." Frédérique stumbles upon a legal, vacant parking space directly outside her building.

Thick wooden double doors open to ancient balustrades, dark slate flooring, and a tiny, metal cage elevator. The lift lurches and rattles along its labored ascent. Squeaking hinges welcome us to Frédérique's apartment and an awaiting bedroom. Down pillows ferry us to sleep.

Sunlight, espresso, and a baguette welcome us back from the dead. A survey of the apartment reveals we spent the night in

Antoine's room. Antoine, Frédérique's eighteen-month-old son, is away on vacation.

"Il est à Nice avec son père," reports Frédérique.

Antoine's crib captures my attention. Its attributes include unfinished wood, a low railing, and vertical slats positioned at four-inch increments. Practical, understated and totally illegal in the United States. Years ago American government scientists determined wide gaps between slats pose mortal danger to infants. If the vertical posts are more than 2 3/8 inches apart, and a baby follows a series of carefully orchestrated movements—left arm here, right foot there—its head could get stuck, resulting in possible choking. The chances of this occurring are one in a million. One, however, is enough for any attorney practicing in the United States.

My eyes continue to scan the room. A modest paper mobile hangs above the illicit crib. It makes no sounds. It does not require eight, double-A, alkaline batteries. It features only a hand-painted, smiling moon. Two stuffed animals rest on a wooden shelf: a brown bear and a green elephant. Neither makes noise when squeezed. Neither walks on its own. Both are simply cotton-filled dolls with button eyes. A blue carpet stretches out across the bedroom floor. A red rubber ball and four wooden cars rest on its low-cut pile.

This is not the baby room of our friends back home. A final inventory of the space uncovers no hulking toy chest, officially licensed toys, baby monitor, SIDS cushion, glider chair, bassinet, or Diaper Genie. There isn't even a Teletubbie.

Vespas, mini-trucks, horns, sirens and bells. The bustling shops of Bienne give way to mountainous terrain. Our Peugot 504, an aging sedan on loan from Francesca's uncle, rattles in fear of a looming, steep descent. Its engine coughs and grumbles as it lumbers up narrow stone roads and hairpin turns. The relentless climb catapults the car's fluttering temperature indicator straight to *Chaud.*

"Allez, Peugeot, allez!" I urge the crippled *voiture.*

Francesca feeds me directions: a left turn, a right, another right, a left after the chalet, another right, and one final left. I park. Our wounded automobile protests the grueling drive with a roar of its rusted cooling fan.

A fragile, yet regal woman clutches a reddish, rosewood cane and sits forward on a nearby bench. A tall, thinning, elegant man stands beside her.

"Grandmaman. Grandpapa." Francesca runs to her grandparents. Each footstep brings her a step closer to childhood. Grandpapa welcomes her with outstretched arms and a firm embrace.

Three days in Switzerland have resurrected Francesca's native French and transformed her physically. *Le, une* and *bonne* move her lips outward, forcing her mouth into a tight circle. The chin juts forward. Angular motion dominates her arms and hands. Francesca tries to share everything with her grandparents during the first minute of their reunion: la grossesse, la nouvelle maison et l'avancement au travail. Grandpapa tells Francesca he wants to visit his favorite country village and enjoy some needed time away from the Home where he and his wife now live.

A turn of the ignition key brings the Peugeot reluctantly back to life. It gathers speed along a bobbing and weaving two-lane road. Orange tractors, stone barns and wire fencing populate the verdant landscape. A traffic signal brings us to a stop. A cow chews its cud. Each movement of its head causes the bell around its neck to clang lazily.

Grandpapa guides us to an austere Protestant chapel.

"Elle a été construite en l'an mille cent cinquante six." He describes the building like a seasoned historian. It takes great effort to translate his perfect, rapid French.

Francesca holds Grandmaman's left arm and guides her up three stone steps. I remember Francesca's grandmother four years ago. She stood upright, her movement slow but deliberate. Her words were vigorous and bright. Now she leans against Francesca, exhausted by the tiny ascent. She struggles to express a thought and curses her weakening grasp of her native tongue. I catch Grandpapa's eye. I see the recognition. The woman he married more than a half century ago is no longer young and vibrant. The body he possessed fifty years earlier is no longer limber and virile. I stare at Francesca. I record her smooth skin and youthful eyes. For a moment, I am ninety years old. My gait slows. My eyes dim.

Francesca's grandfather searches for a favorite restaurant near the church. He finds a shuttered, three-story building. Flowing, worn letters etched above a blockaded entrance suggest this was once a grand eatery.

"C'était un excellent restaurant." He examines the building for the last time. He recalls the meals he ate here. The conversations. The thoughts. The friends. The friends who are no longer.

I park in front of the Home's main entrance. The Peugeot kicks angrily as the flow of gasoline ceases. We follow Francesca's grandparents through a modest lobby, up a flight of stairs, down a hallway and into their rooms. Grandpapa urges us to stand on the private balcony and admire the awe-inspiring view of Bienne and the undulating mountains beyond. He motions for us to sit in the living room. I recognize all the furniture from the chalet that, until a year ago, was their lifelong home. I try to imagine the day when Francesca and I will move our belongings to a retirement community.

I am eighteen sitting with my grandfather in a nursing home. The only piece of furniture in his semi-private room is a hulking hospital bed. He sits slumped in a wheel chair. The smell of urine mixed with ammonia wafts through the hallways. A television blares in the adjacent room. The highly successful and generous man cries softly as his remaining days recede into darkness.

Francesca collapses into tears the moment we leave the parking lot. I can't help but cry, too. I cry for her. I cry for her grandparents. I cry for our own mortality.

The Peugeot huffs and puffs its way up the now familiar mountain road. A second day's worth of rigorous climbing is too much for the four-cylinder beast to bear.

Grandpapa stands in the driveway. Grandmaman sits on a nearby folding chair. I am given directions to an Olympic training center.

We peer inside a large, glass sports complex and watch teenagers practice gymnastics. Young girls in ponytails obediently repeat tumbles, splits and dismounts. Coaches shout encouragement. Grandmaman waits in the car, preferring to avoid the trauma of exiting and re-entering the automobile.

A short hike brings us to an expansive, clay running track. It overlooks a valley speckled with chimneys, spires and trees. Francesca's grandfather watches us imitate world class long-jumpers. Francesca lumbers down a dirt runway and manages no more than a six-inch leap. I don't fare much better. I wonder if Francesca's grandparents did the same fifty years ago.

We sit on an outdoor patio. Wine grapes drape down from above us. Grandpapa wants to treat us to a gourmet meal at his favorite lakeside restaurant.

Pêsche du lac.

Sweet white wine.

Perfect fried potatoes.

Succulent mousse.

Grandpapa urges us to see the boats bobbing just below the patio. As we make our way towards the dock, Francesca's eyes stream with tears.

"I always do this," she says.

We return to the Home and the thrilling private balcony. Francesca tells her grandparents our baby is a boy and his name will be Enrico. Grandpapa gives Francesca a framed drawing and too many Swiss Francs. A heavy, wooden pendulum clock chimes six times.

Francesca embraces her grandmother. "Au revoir, Grandmaman." The moment is so tender neither I, nor Grandpapa, can watch.

Francesca and I descend the Home's main stairway and traverse the lobby. Grandmaman and Grandpapa remain at the top of the stairs. Time stops. Breathing slows. The solar plexus contracts. Our hands rise to say goodbye. We smile bravely. Francesca clutches my arm. She catches her breath.

"Je t'aime!" she calls out to her grandparents. "Je t'aime."

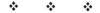

The aging Peugeot lurches down the twisting mountain road. Leaves flutter. Clouds roll. Sunlight dances.

I wonder why life is this way. Why we struggle to fall in love, build a life, and have children only to grow infirm and suffer the pain of old age. The weakened joints. The failing mind. The looming end.

I imagine Enrico's son telling me of the great-grandchild he and his wife are about to have. I imagine Francesca clutching a rosewood cane while I try to recall the name of my daughter-in-law.

Perhaps this is the bargain we all make. In exchange for youth, love and children, we accept old age and its difficult consequences.

Frédérique leads us down a dark side street. We weave between crates, trucks and dumpsters on our way to an abandoned textile factory.

A step inside the cavernous building reveals an unexpected landscape. Elegantly clad people move to and fro underneath blue and green floodlights. A jazz trio explores "Night and Day." Decaying machines reinvent themselves as bars, chairs and sculpture. A waitress leads us to a table and distributes handmade menus. We are in the midst of Geneva's annual artists' festival. Abandoned factories are this year's theme.

In the center of the restaurant twelve children sit at a large table covered with multi-colored clay. An artist moves from one child to another, answering their questions and offering help. I watch various patrons applaud their kids' creations. One boy proudly displays his abstract rendition of an automobile. A girl carefully shapes her clay into a coffee cup. The adults and children coexist effortlessly.

I try to recall seeing anything like this back home. I cannot. In Los Angeles the lives of grownups and children are discrete. Kids do "Kid Things" and adults do "Adult Things." I think of all the lost opportunities generated by this odd American edict.

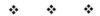

Geneva airport. Au revoirs and tears.
Francesca and I bravely embark on our long journey home.

❖ 5 ❖

No birds chirping. No leaves rustling. No squirrels scurrying. I awaken from a dream whose story I've already forgotten. I wish I could remember all of my dreams, instead of the handful of harrowing ones I'd rather forget. Francesca's recollection is uncanny. No less than three times a week she offers detailed accounts of her unconscious journeys. While I remember a faint color, she recalls the exact texture of a certain phantom's skin. While I recollect in black and white, she reminisces in seventy-millimeter, Dolby Digital, THX Surround.

I roll over onto my side, hoping to catch a glimpse of Francesca's blissful face. I cannot see her face. I cannot see her legs. I cannot see a single inch of her body. All I see is Francesca's hulking pink body pillow.

After shrugging off my initial unease, I thought nothing of the pillow. I actually began to cherish it. Anything that could bring Francesca comfort was welcome in our home. But unease has returned, festered and evolved into something much worse— total dread.

It started innocently enough five days ago. Francesca began referring to the pillow as *him* rather than *it*. A day later she began talking to the rosy intruder saying, "Hi, there" and "I missed you." Yesterday she honored it with a name, Mister Fluffy, as if the pillow deserved to stand alongside other famous Misters like Mister T and the short-lived rock band Mister Mister. Last night Mister Fluffy never left our bed. Tonight is no different. An unapologetic Mister Fluffy lies prone in the center of our mattress, dominating a good third of the Sealy Posturepedic. In forty-eight hours he has become the Great Wall of Pregnancy, dividing Francesca and me into two separate worlds.

I stare at the hulking pink monolith. Francesca's arms wrap tightly around its soft pillowcase and down feathers. I feel wildly insignificant. It's as if I am no longer of value. I have given my sperm, been pushed aside and replaced by Mister Fluffy, the pregnant woman's best friend.

I stare at the ceiling. I leer at the pink whale. "I hate you, Mister Fluffy. I hate you!"

Mister Fluffy snickers, "See? You're talking to me, too."

"Move over," I bark back.

"Sorry, we're fresh out of room over here."

"Jerk."

Francesca stirs. "Honey?"

"Go back to bed," I say.

"Nicely done," Mister Fluffy quips dismissively.

I close my eyes and pray for a swift end to this nightmare.

A spoon bangs against a ceramic bowl. It clatters on the wood floor. Footsteps down the hallway.

"3:40 AM," reports the clock radio.

Francesca stands in the doorway. "I'm having cereal," she says. "I woke up and thought cereal."

The microwave oven beeps. Its door slams shut. Footsteps down the hallway.

"4:45 AM," reports the clock radio.

"I'm having a frozen burrito," she says. "I woke up and thought burrito."

The refrigerator compressor rattles. The freezer door slams shut. Footsteps down the hallway.

"5:50 AM," reports the clock radio.

"I'm having a scoop of Coffee Heath Bar Crunch," she says. "I woke up and thought Coffee Heath Bar Crunch."

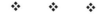

The starter motor wines. The engine roars. No footsteps down the hallway.

"6:23 AM," reports the clock radio.

I sit up. My ultimate nightmare has come true. I am alone in bed with Mister Fluffy.

Large blue placards scream out from every angle. STROLLERS. CRIBS. TOYS. BASSINETS.

Hundreds of doped shoppers speed past one another, avoiding collisions by the narrowest of margins. Young children drag behind their parents, sighing at every turn. Defeated employees in bright blue smocks ricochet from one crazed customer to another. Sky-high ceilings and endless shelving stretch out as far as the eye can see. A sense of awe, a wave of religiosity overwhelms us as we struggle to comprehend this cathedral of newborn consumerism. BabysRUs. *Temple of gestation. Mecca of reproduction. Church of the expectant.*

A grinning sales associate offers us a *Baby Basics* checklist and a bar code reader straight from "Star Wars." In spite of its densely spaced, microscopic print, the checklist fills both sides of a pale blue, 8 x 11 flyer. It bubbles with the mysterious words. *Onesie. Footsie. Layette. Teether.*

"What's a layette?" I ask.

"Something a newborn needs," Francesca replies wisely.

A wall of humidifiers confronts me with an unimaginable selection of features, the benefits of which elude me: *Medicine Dispensing Reservoir. Ultrasonic. Dual Timer. High Output. Vaporizer. Slant/Fin Germ Free.* Only faint memories of my childhood humidifier offer possible clues: white metal base, musty odor, long black electrical cord, transparent plastic dome filled with bubbling water and steam wafting out a circular opening at the top. A percolating Pantheon of Vapor. I do not remember any timers, filters, flashing lights, or even an on-off switch. Obviously the world of steam has evolved into an advanced science based on exotic theorems and breakthrough research.

An expectant mother in a wheelchair rolls up beside me. "Excuse me," she asks. "Do you know the difference between ultrasonic and non-ultrasonic humidifiers?" I want to kiss her. I want to hug her. I am not the only one.

"I have no idea," I confess.

"You looked like you did."

"I'm a professional actor."

An endless line of strollers welcomes me to Aisle 7. Milano XL. Pliko Matic. Opus IV. LiteRider. CitiSport. A Venezia taunts me with its elegant Italian styling. I approach the carriage cautiously, acutely aware I'm entering more uncharted territory. Initial examination uncovers two plastic foot switches labeled 1 and 2, and two unmarked hand switches. Instincts tell me the chair somehow collapses. I press switches 1 and 2 believing they will trigger a miraculous folding sequence. The Venezia refuses to budge. I turn the chair on its side, hoping to find a fifth switch labeled *Hidden Master Release*. Careful examination reveals nothing of the kind. I click the numbered switches again and add the hand switches to the mix. Venezia remains frozen in place, taunting me with its rigidity. I begin to suspect scientists have made me their unwitting subject in a perverse, undercover intelligence test, lowering my score with each failed attempt. I throw all four switches into random positions and try my luck again. The stroller strains and twists against the full force of my muscles. My score drops to 3, the numeric equivalent of moron. I surrender to the rolling Rubik's Cube, place it back in its display rack and slither away, defeated.

"I will return" is my silent vow. "I will return."

In spite of my failure, I take pride in knowing more about baby carriages than ever before. I now know they are sophisticated, hi-tech devices, not to be mocked. I know they require extensive, hands-on training and, in a matter of months, will probably boast low impact air-bags and eight-speaker stereo sound.

I flash on Antoine's stroller. No American would dare purchase it. It doesn't have built-in safety straps or a dual seatbelt anchoring system. It has no extended footrest cushion or optional skull pillow. It is only a chair designed to transport a baby.

"What do you think of the crib bumpers?" asks Francesca.

"Huh?"

I turn left onto ACTIVITY CENTER Avenue. A green plastic Snuggly Car jiggles on top of bright yellow springs. Its dashboard overflows with buttons, horns and bells. An apple red Megasaucer sports music maker, teethers, a steering wheel, a central padded seat, and the ability to twist and turn. It looks like the bridge of a miniature Starship Enterprise.

"Kids love these," says Francesca.

"I didn't know they even existed," I quip, wondering if an adult version of this spinning saucer could start some sort of new fad. Distraught executives might discover rotating clockwise while grooving to "London Bridges" induces better concentration. People might flock to discos and whirl in giant plastic orbs, bouncing off one another like erotic, spinning tops.

"Megasaucer or Snuggly Car?" I ask.

"The Megasaucer looks too big for our living room," observes Francesca. She's right. The moment the saucer landed, a couch or coffee table would have to go.

I wave the Star Wars bar-code reader across the roadster's UPC tag.

"Evenflo Snuggly Car," announces the liquid crystal display.

Another wall of glossy boxes. Another enormous blue sign. BABY MONITORS. *Two Channel. Hi-Power 900mhz Output. Graphic LCD display. Digital Volume Control.* I wonder what parents did before infant monitors existed. Perhaps a baby's cries actually traveled from the newborn's throat, out its mouth, down a hallway, through a bedroom door and into the parent's ears. Perhaps, mothers and fathers simply *heard* their children's cries.

"Signal Scrambler," announces a splashy blue and yellow carton.

I imagine a white panel van parked outside our house. Inside the unassuming vehicle a spy intercepts and unscrambles our baby's encoded cries. He lustily e-mails the translated message:

FROM: Secret Agent

TO: HQ
SUBJECT: Herman Baby

Message as follows:
Goo-goo.
Ga-ga.

Please advise.

The baby registry desk stands before us. We collapse into chairs, exhausted by our four-hour journey through BabysRUs. A pimply sales associate plugs the barcode reader into a computer and downloads our selections. Francesca removes a shoe and rubs a blistered, bright red foot.

"Sir," asks the adolescent salesman, "do you want baby shower insert cards or standard cards?"

"What?"

"They're free."

"What's free?"

"The cards or inserts."

"Yes, I'll take them."

"Which? The cards or inserts?"

"Yes.

Orange red clouds roll past receding rays of sunlight. The moon prepares to relieve its daytime counterpart. I rest my backpack on the foyer floor and exhale a day's worth of auditions, traffic, and smog.

The din of television lures me down the hallway. A mind-numbing MTV recess seems like just the remedy for a mediocre day. As I approach the open bedroom door, I see my wife's feet, ankles, and then...nothing more. An expansive patch of pink obscures the remainder of her body. I contemplate the scene: Francesca and her constant compadre locked in an embrace. A creaking floorboard startles them both. I search Francesca's watery eyes and Mister Fluffy's wide grin.

"Hi," says Francesca on the verge of tears.

"It's about time," Mister Fluffy admonishes me. I suppress a sudden impulse to strangle the pink interloper. I remind myself that Mister Fluffy is no more than down feathers and cotton.

"The baby kicked all day." Francesca rubs her stomach in a slow circular pattern. "Work was a total disaster. Mary wants out by January, the factory pressed a faulty master, Todd's on jury duty and Larry's vacation started today."

I push Mister Fluffy aside and massage Francesca's shoulders. The body pillow grunts in disgust.

"Now I have to hire another director and create a new organizational structure." Francesca wipes her nose with Kleenex. Even in the notoriously chaotic music business this is beyond the realm.

The television flickers with images of a sickly woman and a cello. I recognize the film, "Hillary and Jackie," the story of a world class cellist who contracts multiple sclerosis and dies at forty-two. Not ideal viewing for a depressed, pregnant woman. Perhaps "Bambi" would be a better choice. Uplifting music. A lovable deer. Thumper the Rabbit. I flash on the movie's conclusion and reconsider. A forest fire. Death. Bambi the orphan. Suddenly the heartwarming children's classic seems more like "The Shining."

Jackie stares at the cello she can no longer play. She feels herself receding from the life she once knew. The life she once controlled. She clutches the armrest of her wheelchair. Francesca clutches my hand.

"I feel like I'm losing control," she says. "Like everything is beyond my reach."

Jackie slumps in her chair. Francesca slumps under the covers. The bedside alarm clock clicks one second after another.

"Touch my stomach."

I place my palms on Francesca's abdomen. Enrico kicks and moves in every direction imaginable. What were once faint taps are now distinct thuds. What were once slight movements are now hardy somersaults. A bulge crests in Francesca's mid-section sending a tremor through her body. My wife has become California and Enrico the San Andreas Fault.

"Do you see how much pain I'm in? He's kicking all the time."

"At least he's kicking. Lots of women panic if their babies don't kick."

Francesca's scowl tells me I've just failed the compassion test. "A little panic wouldn't be so bad right now," she says. "Anything's better than nonstop aches."

I wisely change my tact. "This must be really hard for you."

"It is." A fierce punch emanates from Francesca's bellybutton. My hand recoils in shock. "Did you feel that?"

"Yes. Absolutely." I wonder how anyone within fifty feet could miss it.

"No, you didn't."

"I did."

"Open your mouth."

"What?"

"Do it."

I surrender to my wife's crazed request.

"This is what it feels like." With a firm outstretched finger Francesca jabs my right, inner cheek. "Now you know what it's like," she crosses her arms and grunts.

I search for another antidote to her misery. "Imagine yourself on a beautiful Hawaiian beach," I whisper. "Palm trees swaying. Waves crashing."

"Ugh!" Francesca reels from a swift, merciless jab. She rolls away from me, grabs Mister Fluffy, and prays for relief.

"Everything will be alright," Mister Fluffy assures her.

Francesca's eyes close. Her breathing eases. Peace.

I reconsider my pink foe. I realize Mister Fluffy is not my nemesis. He is and always has been a Good Samaritan. Someone who expects nothing in return for his tireless efforts. I feel an awkward sense of regret.

"Nice job." My first peace offering.

"I was born to do this," replies Mister Fluffy.

A silence.

"By the way," he continues.

"What?"

"Don't get too jealous. She'll toss me aside like yesterday's news when Enrico arrives."

"That's not true, Mister Fluffy." I feel a twinge of guilt. It's as if I have betrayed an old friend. "You'll always be part of the family," I promise him.

"Trust me," he replies stoically, "I'll be in the blue recycle bin by February."

"I'm so sorry."

"It's the price you pay for riding so high."

Mister Fluffy. The Icarus of Pregnancy.

Another silence.

"Well, I'm glad you're here."

"Thanks," Mister Fluffy's voice cracks ever so slightly. "That means a lot to me."

Seven AM. The clock radio wrestles us out of bed.

"How did you sleep?" I ask.

"Really well." Francesca smiles.

I bury my head under a pillow. An infinitely empty day stretches before me. No appointments. No auditions. No jobs.

Francesca rockets out of bed, suits up, and bounds out the front door. Have a great day!" she hollers.

"You, too," I grumble.

I roll onto my side and consider Plato, our teddy bear and resident philosopher. He leans against a copy of Nabokov's *The Eye* and ponders some unknown, complex hypothesis.

"What am I doing?" I ask.

The furry philosopher contemplates my nondescript inquiry, scratches his nose and stares searchingly into my eyes. "I have no idea," he concludes.

"That's it?" I ask, expecting a grand revelation.

"That's it."

Plato returns to his thoughts.

Six months and counting. Twelve weeks to go. Childhood memories rush forward.

My mother and I buying vegetables in Chinatown. "Would you like an egg roll, Perry?"

The Ernie hand puppet my parents bought at a Berkeley crafts fair.

Marching for peace down a wide boulevard.

My father lifting me over a balustrade. "I can see the street below," I say, struggling to mask my overwhelming fear.

The army green, Smith-Corona typewriter I used to write stories about talking penguins, a benevolent queen, and an elk that could not find his mother.

Raggedy Anns and Andys. Each with its own name, personality and voice.

My Fischer-Price garage. My Fischer-Price town. My Fischer-Price airport.

Building a scale model of the Golden Gate Bridge. My brother rigging twine to create a true suspension bridge. "See how the middle arches upwards?"

Hurling books across my room in the midst of a temper tantrum.

Sitting on the toilet with the door open, my father urging me on, singing the "Doo-Wack-A-Doo" song.

Making paper cutouts of gondolas and ski areas.

Standing in the driveway of my summer camp. Weeping as my parents drive away.

Standing in the driveway of my summer camp. Weeping as my parents return. "Summer's over."

Hugging my grandfather, Pam-Pam.

Fenway Park. Box seats. "Pam-Pam, can I have some popcorn?"

Listening to a Red Sox's radio broadcast while torrential rain batters shuttered storm windows.

Sitting in the hallway of my elementary school. Banished, once again, for insubordination.

Doing the box step with Helen M—.

Lying on my father's lap—the signal for a long back scratch.

Leaping onto my mother's leg, grabbing hold of her ankle and becoming the Leg Leach.

Kissing Lisa B—at my eighth grade dance.

My brother and I exploring Golden Gate Park, making secret trails and eating Japanese seaweed crackers.

Seeing my first story published in a children's magazine.

Standing next to Lee Grant on a movie set.

Reading *Peanuts* anthologies from cover to cover. "I'm just like Linus," I think.

Las Vegas and the Grand Canyon.

My parents screaming at each other. Doors crashing shut. Angry footsteps pounding across floorboards.

The unfinished spiral staircase. The staircase that my father was going to complete.

Dad's one-bedroom apartment. Our first meal together as single men.

Mother and I eating in an empty house.

Meeting my father's first girlfriend.

Meeting my mother's first girlfriend.

Drinking gin and tonics in high school.

Watching other people date.

Watching too much television.

Vomiting in a sink.

A Berkeley dorm room. My roommate's pungent Kim Chi.

Getting a blow job at three in the morning from a girl I hardly know.

Obsessing about exams.

Worrying about everything.

Drinking anything.

Transferring to an East Coast college.

"Your grandfather passed away last night."

Standing before a sealed, wooden coffin.

Meeting a hall mate.

Meeting his girlfriend.

"Hi," she says.

"Hi," I respond.

"Perry?"

"Yes?"

"I'm Francesca."

"Francesca?"

My wife to be. The mother of my child.

What will Enrico's story be?

Glistening stars against a jet-black sky confirm the ungodly hour of 5 AM. The Boston wedding of Francesca's college roommate forces us, once again, back on the road. As I struggle with two reluctant, rolling suitcases, Francesca wavers under the weight of an overstuffed, orange backpack. We rest the luggage against the Maxima's rear bumper and review our standard travel checklist.

"Toothbrushes?"

"Check!"

"Underwear?"

"Check!"

"Sweaters?"

Silence.

We scamper into the house, collect two wool sweaters and toss them into a shopping bag. Francesca and I hurry back to the car and resume the checklist.

"Sneakers?"

"Check!"

"Dress Shoes?"

"Check!"

"Bridesmaid dress?"

Silence.

We throw open the front door, plow through our chaotic closets and stuff Francesca's satin dress and my suit—also forgotten—into a voluminous canvas sack.

"Hats?"

"Check!"

"Money?"

"Check!"

"Tickets?"

"Check!"

The car roars to life and slowly backs into the street. Francesca adjusts the heating vents and stereo controls.

"Stop!" screams Francesca. My foot slams on the brake pedal. Tires squeal. The car lurches forward. Eyes dart, looking for an injured dog or cat. Nothing but the empty roads stretches out before us.

"Mister Fluffy!"

"What?" I ask in disbelief.

"I forgot Mister Fluffy."

"You want to bring Mister Fluffy?"

Francesca's door slams shut in reply. My wife disappears into the darkness. A minute later she returns triumphantly with the pink monolith. Even in the darkness I can see Mister Fluffy's grin.

"Anything else?" I check my watch to see if our flight has already left.

Mister Fluffy bobs down the narrow aisles of the 767 wide-body. Passengers stare in disbelief, praying they won't soon be his seatmate. We locate 27A and 27B. 27C, a dour, pinstripe suited man, sighs in defeat. I buckle myself in and peruse the familiar *Sky Emporium* catalog. Francesca explores various positions hoping one will bring comfort. Left side leaning against the seatback. Legs curled around her down-filled companion. Body slumped low in the chair.

"There." Francesca's movements stop.

"Cozy?" I ask, my words muffled by Mister Fluffy, whose upper torso presses firmly against my face.

"Yes, thank you."

I try to tolerate my predicament, knowing Francesca has finally found comfort. I turn my head sideways, a successful tactic until 27C demands I stop breathing in his ear. I push Mister Fluffy aside. He pops back instantly. A scuffle ensues, and in the midst of landing a left jab, I mistakenly elbow 27C.

"Sorry," I apologize.

The forty-something man replies with a cold stare. "I'm tired," say his hollow eyes. "Don't touch me."

I wedge Mister Fluffy under my right arm and immobilize him. I relish my emancipation until Francesca shifts unexpectedly. Her movement frees Mister Fluffy and launches him, once again, on a collision course with my nose. I instinctively recoil and brush up against 27C.

"That's enough," declares the morose businessman. He abandons his seat in favor of 35E.

I seize the moment and buckle Mister Fluffy into the newly vacant chair.

The jetliner lumbers down the runway and begins the miraculous feat of lifting into the thin air.

"Can you get me headphones?" asks Mister Fluffy.

"You're lucky you're not in the luggage compartment," I snap. "They don't heat the luggage compartment."

I'm certain I hear Mister Fluffy gulp.

The pink obelisk sleeps soundly as we soar over Denver.

"Should I call the other agents and tell them to hold off a bit longer? This is so fucked!"

"Stop swearing, Perry. Every other word out of your mouth is fuck."

"It's just that this is so unfair. My agent is supposed to work for *me*. I hired him, not the other way around. How much more does my career have to suffer before he'll release me? Listen to me! *Release me*. What am I, a slave? An indentured servant? I tell you everyone just wants to screw actors. We're just these poor suckers caught in the middle of self-serving agents and greedy producers. Why do I do this? Why? I could have become an attorney."

"You hate lawyers."

"I should've stayed with database programming. I could have ended up with some Internet thing and become a millionaire."

"Perry?"

"What?"

"Did you ever think your anxiety has something to do with Enrico's impending arrival?"

"Maybe."

"Let me assure you, it does." Francesca rubs my arm.

"My agent is a real fuck—"

"—Yes, Perry."

"Maybe this vacation will be good for me."

"Maybe it will."

I consider the slumbering Mister Fluffy and his simple life. No worries. No troubles. No bills to pay. I find myself yearning for a similar existence, a reprieve from the endlessly uncertain freelance life.

A thought derails the dream: The blue recycle bin.

Francesca and I race across Government Center's expansive brick plaza. We brave a boulevard teeming with unpredictable Boston drivers and dash into the Oyster House. Francesca's best friend, the bride-to-be, welcomes us with her trademark sarcasm, "You finally made it."

New England clam chowder, soft-shell Maine lobster, white wine and a Tiffany's gift bag populate our table. Francesca peeks inside the bag and discovers a pair of elegant silver earrings. A young couple approaches us.

"This is Grace and I'm Ian," offers the husband.

"Nice to meet you," I reciprocate.

"Looks like we're table mates," he says, referring to a seating placard. Grace rubs her rounded abdomen in the telltale "I'm pregnant" fashion.

"How far along are you?" asks Francesca between bites of butter-filled lobster meat.

"Three and a half months. How about you?"

"Six."

Ian and I drink wine. Francesca and Grace make do with sparkling water.

"We just started decorating the baby's room," confesses Grace.

"Don't worry," I chuckle. "We haven't done anything." My stomach drops. I can't believe we've ignored something so crucial.

Grace tells us her uterus is heart-shaped. "I'm a little scared because it means the baby will be born premature."

"But, with all the machines and techniques available now," pipes in Ian, "everything should be okay."

"Thank God for modern medicine," adds Grace.

I think about modern medicine a lot. Less than a hundred years ago pregnancy often ended in hemorrhaging, infection and death. I can't imagine losing Francesca. Our life has just begun.

The rehearsal dinner comes to a close. Ian and Grace wish us luck and disappear into a crowd of people. Francesca and I brace ourselves for the icy air outside.

The setting sun drenches the wedding reception in blinding, golden light. Crystal champagne chalices clink. Caterers ferry appetizers from one guest to another. Partygoers share stories about the bride and groom. Francesca holds court next to the bar, surrounded by her college roommates and their husbands.

"We need a picture of this," she decides.

The women stand in a neat row, their smiles bathed in sunlight. The husbands line up behind them, their faces cast in shadow. A stranger offers to take the photo. I grasp Francesca's waist and gaze into the lens.

"Smile!" commands the unknown cameraman.

Only twelve years separate us all from our college graduations. In that time we have built careers, fallen in love, married, bought homes and started families. A blink of an eye and we approach middle age. The hour hand whirs.

Orange flames fall from bare branches. Aging lobster boats, abandoned for the winter, bob to and fro. Circling gulls scan the choppy surf for dinner. Icy wind bores through my jacket, sweater, turtleneck, undershirt and skin. Francesca and her mother, Laure, walk ahead, their silhouettes framed by evergreens and naked birches.

"Remember when I used to dress Puffy and Pumpkin in scarves and hats?" Francesca recalls her childhood cats. "Then I'd photograph them in front of an Hawaiian backdrop."

We pass a neighbor's house. Inside, an elderly man laments his wife's death. Three years have passed and yet her voice remains on the answering machine's outgoing message.

"Puffy and Pumpkin used to spend afternoons there," remembers Francesca. "I used to come looking for them."

A twelve-year old Francesca sprints down the street calling out, "Puffy? Pumpkin?"

"They're right here," shouts the cheerful lobsterman's wife.

Francesca returns home, her feline companions in tow. Laure welcomes the brood with a smile. Her face of twenty years ago looks just Francesca's face today.

Salmon steaks, potatoes, bread, salad, and baked squash decorate the dining table. Brown speckles glisten in the squashes' orange innards, the promise of Vermont maple syrup.

The kitchen's rotary dial telephone clangs to life. Its vigorous metal clapper broadcasts a harsh ring throughout the house.

"Hallo?" Twenty-five years of American living cannot diminish Laure's native, Swiss-French accent. "It's for you, Francesca."

"I'll take it in the den." Francesca grabs a binder filled with notes, telephone numbers and manufacturing data.

"If we were on Mars, she'd still get calls from her office," I quip as I delve into a succulent piece of salmon.

Francesca returns too quickly.

"I failed my glucose check," she announces. "Doctor Braintree says I scored two hundred and one at the two-hour mark."

"What does that mean?"

"It means I have gestational diabetes."

I flash on Jeremy, high school friend and juvenile diabetic, who regularly injected himself with insulin. I remember being thankful not to have to do the same. I recall my grandmother warning my grandfather not to eat too much sugar. I remember my grandfather sneaking cheese blintzes at the International House of Pancakes. "Don't tell your grandmother," he would say. "It's our secret."

"What happens now?" I ask.

"More tests when we return home."

Gestational diabetes. Something *other* pregnant women get. The ones you don't know. The ones you read about. My wife.

Francesca's father and I sit together at the now empty dining table. He examines a medical reference book, a remnant of his recent general practitioner days. He locates a dense passage and embarks on a simple sketch of the bloodstream. Six squares with rounded edges line up inside two parallel lines. Six cells inside a vein.

"Cells absorb glucose and use it to power the body. The cells are semi-permeable which means they can't absorb glucose unless insulin is present. If the body isn't producing enough insulin, the bloodstream floods with glucose."

"And a flood of glucose causes diabetes?" I ask.

"It can create diabetic symptoms."

"Is that what two-hundred and one represents?"

"Yes."

"What should Francesca do?"

"She has to carefully monitor sugar intake. That means avoiding carbohydrate-rich foods like pasta, bread, and cereal." He has just named Francesca's three, all-time favorite foods in descending order. For Francesca, a world without pasta is a world without oxygen. A world without bread is a world without water. A world without Sugar Corn Pops just isn't a world.

I retire to my wife's high school bedroom. Francesca sleeps fitfully, her arms clenched tightly around Mister Fluffy. I kiss her forehead. She shifts slightly. Her frown relaxes into a smile.

Breakfast. I guiltily spread strawberry jam onto a thick egg bagel. Francesca stares longingly at the mega-carbohydrate.

"You want some orange juice?" I ask.

"What do you think?" Francesca jabs a fork into a scoop of cottage cheese.

"Sorry," I backpedal. "How about some water?"

"How about it?" The blunt reply.

"Nothing. It's just here. In case you want it. In this pitcher. That's all."

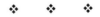

I stuff a final shopping bag into the tiny trunk of my brother's metallic blue Beetle. I sprint up the back staircase and into the kitchen. I find Francesca and Laure embracing. Tears stream from their eyes.

"I love you, Mom."

"I love you, too." Laure struggles against the sorrow.

Francesca hugs her father. He brushes away a teardrop and kisses her cheek. A lifetime of strife momentarily vanishes. Decades of tempers, rebellion and silence recede into a distant horizon, replaced by the promise of a grandson.

The Beetle backs out of the driveway and accelerates down the main road. Francesca's parents wave to us from the garage. I stare into the rearview mirror and watch their bodies shrink into indistinct shapes.

Midnight nears. Francesca sleeps soundly. My brother Daniel, his wife, Kate, and I sit around a low, black matte coffee table. Stainless steel shelves, dimmed halogen lights and trip-hop music surround us.

"This is my last year of teaching," proclaims Kate. Decades of formal education have taken their toll. A doctorate of history represents both a stunning achievement and a depressing reminder of years lost to academia.

"I spend zillions of hours preparing lectures and grading papers." Kate considers a mound of class notes on the dining table. "I get nothing back. I mean, I love my students, but I can't keep doing this. I'm being paid nothing. I have to supervise two teaching assistants. I do all this work and, yet, I have no hope of tenure. Plus, the ultimate curse, I'm a woman. My department is one giant fraternity." She fidgets with her wristwatch. "I don't know what I'm going to after this summer. Do I write my book? Do I work for some company? Who's going to hire a Ph.D.?"

Kate's predicament strikes a cord. The uncertainty. The need to do something substantial and worthwhile with one's life. The need to *amount to something.*

"My education will be wasted if I don't publish something." She spins a silver bangle around her wrist. "I always think about arriving, coming to the place when my life starts and finally has meaning."

I've spent a lifetime awaiting my arrival, the moment when I would feel fully realized. I used to think I would arrive when I completed my first guest star on television. When I did, I felt no closer to arriving. When I booked a huge national advertising campaign, arrival still eluded me.

"Maybe you never arrive." My thought lands somewhere between the three of us. "Maybe life is simply about having kids, being great parents and dying. Maybe everything else is just noise."

"Maybe," says Kate. "But I've judged my whole life in terms of career. I feel like I've done nothing. And, if we have a kid, I won't have any time to finish what I've started. I'm thirty-six."

"It's so weird when you think how short life is," I remark.

"I'm scared of death," adds Kate.

My body turns ice cold. I can't move. My breathing halts. *I'm really going to die.* The thought cuts me to the core. Someday soon my heart will stop beating, and I will be no more. I will die. Francesca will die. Enrico will die. We will all die. In a few thousand days, the end.

"Okay, I'm officially freaking out." I pace the room. "Complete and total terror right now."

"Me too!" Kate joins in my anxious march. "Turn on the lights, Daniel. Turn them on now!"

The previously dim halogen lamps blaze brightly.

"Better?" My brother leans against the light switch. A slight, but noticeable smile creeps across his face.

"Yes, thanks," I snip, failing to see any humor in death.

"Good." Daniel stands before a cluttered kitchen sink and begins washing the night's dishes.

I am struck by my brother's assuredness. It occurs to me that his architectural career and lifelong soul-searching have created an undeniable sense of arrival. Massive, immutable buildings of his design undisputedly establish his existence. Coherent beliefs about reincarnation and the soul clarify his relationship with mortality and God.

I don't know what I believe. My relationship with God and death is uncertain. When I found myself in the midst of the San Francisco earthquake, I discovered that I believe in God. "God, please let me live," I pleaded as I crouched beneath an office desk. But what God? God, the benevolent force? God, the white-haired king of heaven? God, the all-loving earth mother?

I climb a dark staircase to the upstairs floor and ease open the front bedroom door. As my pupils widen, the outline of

Francesca's abdomen becomes clear. I think about Enrico inside. I hope he is well. I pray he will develop normally. I pray I will be a good father. I pray. I pray to a God I do not know.

What will I tell Enrico when he asks me about death? What will I tell Enrico when he asks me about God?

My father holds a white railing in place while I struggle to attach it to an unfinished crib.

"You want the bolts to go in the top hole," Cousin Ralph explains. "When Enrico gets bigger, you'll use the lower hole."

"Top hole," I confirm. "Got it." My hand grips a tiny Allen wrench. With each quarter turn of the tool, my fingers slam into the crib frame "Dammit!" A knuckle starts to bleed.

"Cut yourself?" asks Ralph.

"Yup."

"I remember this part wasn't too easy."

We are reassembling the crib used by my cousin's boys during their infant years. I remember peering through the white railing and singing them to sleep.

"Fuck!" Another laceration.

A final turn of the bolt. Three generations of fathers step back to admire their work.

"Looks pretty good," observes my dad.

"Just like new!" pipes in Ralph.

"I'm really going to be a parent," I blurt. The finished crib eliminates any remaining illusions about still being a single guy on the prowl.

"Don't worry," Ralph rubs my shoulder. "You'll do great." I'm certain I detect a deep sense of relief in his voice. I can feel him saying, "Thank God it's not me. I don't have the energy any more."

I place my elbows on the front railing and imagine Enrico peering up at me. In an instant the railing crashes downward, sending my body straight towards the unmerciful hardwood floor.

"The railing is adjustable." Cousin Ralph slides the bar up and down. "See?"

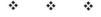

Francesca and I find comfort in the familiar surroundings of our obstetrician's office: the wooden golden retriever standing guard, prescription glasses scattered everywhere, academic plaques covering the walls.

"I may have to leave at any moment. A patient is about to give birth." Doctor Braintree quickly reviews Francesca's chart. "I want to see you again next week. We're going to have to meet more often because of your condition."

An excited nurse bounds into the room. "She's fully dilated."

"I'm referring you to a specialist. He'll determine if diet modification can control your diabetes. If not, you'll have to take insulin." The doctor grabs his mask. "Sorry. Got to go."

We exit the office without a saying a word. A straight path with one right turn carries us past exam rooms, the reception area and into a lifeless, gray building lobby.

Francesca fights an onslaught of tears. "He said I have a *condition.*"

Neither of us has the courage to venture beyond the lobby's main area. Instead, we settle into a pair of uncomfortable plastic chairs and stare at two unremarkable paintings. A coyote howling at the moon. Waves crashing against a generic seashore.

Stained beige carpet. Clumsy furniture. Flickering fluorescent light. Francesca approaches a faux marble reception counter.

"I'm here for diabetes counseling," she tells a bored office assistant.

"The doctor will be right with you" is the mechanical reply.

A cheap desk clock marks one second after another. It soon devours ten minutes of our lives.

Realizing that "right with you" actually means "wait," we delve into a pile of outdated magazines, hoping one will keep us occupied. *Bazaar. Cosmopolitan. Ladies Home Journal.* No luck.

My attention shifts to a wall calendar, obviously the gift of some pharmaceutical sales rep. Its black and white date grid is dwarfed by huge green letters spelling Zoloxiphine, a name only drug company lexicographers could create. I try to imagine what this breakthrough drug does. Combat depression? Cure diabetes? Improve sexual performance? I settle on appetite control.

With the Zoloxiphine mystery solved, I scan the room for additional entertainment and settle on the pockmarked ceiling tiles above me. I start the count. One. Two. Three.

Twenty more minutes vanish into a sea of lost time. I reconsider *Ladies Home Journal.*

"Go right ahead," drones a lobotomized receptionist.

An exam table draped in quilted, pink paper draws Francesca into its uncomfortable, rigid clutches. The paper sheet does nothing to remedy the table's unforgiving, flattened cushions.

"Do you know the sex of the baby?" asks a cheerful, freckled sonogram operator.

"That's not why we're here," I answer brusquely. The technician recoils, her mouth droops.

Francesca's face fills with embarrassment. "She's just finding out if we already know. That's all."

"Oh." I offer the woman a sheepish smile. I notice the name Mandy etched on her name badge. "Sorry. I guess I'm a little edgy."

"Everything's going to be alright," Mandy assures us.

Two computer screens flicker to life and in an instant I see Enrico. A head. A nose. Fingers. A spine. A complete body floating inside Francesca's uterus.

"How is everything? Is everything alright?" the words spurt from my mouth.

"Looks like a healthy brain. Placenta has a good amount of fluid. Your baby's doing great."

My back straightens. The shoulders relax. The neck releases.

Mandy leads us across a narrow hallway and into a cramped office. Official looking certificates blanket the tiny room's walls. *Cums, lauds* and *magnas* punctuate the framed credentials. Francesca and I sit patiently in bulky, wooden captain's chairs. Minutes pass. I examine a conspicuously positioned photograph of a grinning family and its dog. I check my watch. Another ten minutes disappear.

"Where is he?" I ask.

"Beats me." Francesca's voice is laced with frustration.

We wait another five minutes.

"Maybe he's at lunch."

"Maybe he's dead."

A sudden turn of a doorknob announces the arrival of our specialist. He breezes past us, takes his place behind a cluttered desk, and adjusts his standard issue, white lab coat. An embroidered breast pocket patch introduces us to Doctor Shell.

Doctor Shell examines Francesca's glucose test results. "These numbers are very high. If diet doesn't work, you're going to have to take insulin." *Insulin.* "I'm referring you to a diabetes clinic. They'll discuss proper nutrition and explain how to use a glucose monitor." His monotone speech pattern does little to calm us. "You're going to have to check your sugar level every four hours."

"Every four hours," Francesca repeats.

The doctor's attention shifts to a mound of manila folders strewn across his desk. He sorts them into a series of neat piles. The meaning of each stack eludes me.

"Can we ask some questions?" I ask, sensing the doctor has already left the room.

"Fire away," he answers offhandedly.

"Does exercise have any impact on Francesca's condition?"

"Exercise is always great." Doctor Shell glances at Francesca. "Are you exercising?"

"I'm walking in the morning," she offers.

"A stroll or a more vigorous walk?"

"Stroll."

"Limited, more vigorous exercise would be better." He springs from his chair, folders in hand, and bolts for the door. "If you need anything else, feel free to call." The doctor disappears down the hallway.

"Is that it?" I ask dumbfounded. "Where'd he go?"

"I guess to his next patient."

We trudge back to the front desk.

"Uh," I sputter, "the doctor is referring us to a diabetes clinic of some kind."

"We'll call you once the paperwork is processed," replies the blank receptionist.

"When will that be?"

"We'll call you."

End of conversation.

Thick traffic and the setting sun. My attention moves from the road where it should be to my cellular phone where it shouldn't.

"Hello?" I barely miss slamming into a Chevy Astro, the third near collision of the day. "Yes, my wife Francesca...F-R-A-N-C-E-S-C-A. No...F-R-A-N...Yes, that's it..." I dodge a stalled Mercedes M320. "Doctor Shell referred my wife to you. She needs diabetes counseling. Yes...That's right...Next Friday? No, she has gestational diabetes. She needs to see you right away."

A stoplight, the driver's cellular sanctuary.

"Let me give you my pager number. Maybe if you have a cancellation or something..."

A car horn blares behind me, the traffic signal beams green.

"I called yesterday about diabetes counseling for my wife Francesca...F-R-A-N-C-E-S-C-A." I fiddle with the winding, black cord that connects my cell phone to the cigarette lighter. "Yes, that's her. Do you have any appointments available today or tomorrow?"

Hold music. Goo Goo Dolls. *"...reruns become our history..."*

"Next Friday? No, she has gestational diabetes. She must see you right away."

Hold music. Elton John. *"...the circle of life, the..."*

"Let me give you my pager number. Maybe if you have a cancellation or something...Hello?"

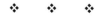

"Hi, I called last week. My wife has gestational diabetes and…"

Hold music. Backstreet Boys. *"…the shape of my heart…"*

"Okay…Is Friday still available? No?"

Hold music. Backstreet Boys. *"…the shape of my heart…"*

I stare at the digital display hoping for a low number, something less than one hundred.

"Eighty-six," flashes the screen.

"That's good. Right?" I ask the nurse administering the glucose test.

"I'm not a diabetes specialist," she answers diplomatically, "but it seems within normal range."

Francesca downs six ounces of orange-flavored glucose. The second phase of the test begins.

"I'll check your sugar levels in one hour," explains the nurse. "In the meantime, you can wait in the lobby."

Francesca and I review the available publications brimming from a simulated wood magazine rack: *Parenting. Parents. Working Mother. American Baby. Highlights.* I grab a periodical and leaf through its glossy pages:

Although a baby sleeps sixteen to twenty hours a day, she awakes often, leaving the parent with no time to get any real sleep. (p. 10)

Expect to be exhausted for the first two months. (p. 32)

Some babies reverse day and night, causing a very challenging sleeping environment. (p. 57)

Be sure to pick the right diaper bag. (p. 42)

I reach for *Highlights,* hoping it will carry me through the remaining wait period. *Goofus plays with matches. Galant finds a matchbook and asks his mother to put it in a safe place.* I hate Galant.

The nurse pricks Francesca's finger once more. We stare at the liquid crystal display and pray for a low number.

"One hundred ninety," blinks the screen.

"Is that a good number?" I ask, sensing the answer is "No."

"You'll have to talk to the doctor," the nurse replies kindly.

Doctor Braintree examines the results.

I break the excruciating silence, "Is one-ninety good?"

"No. It's very elevated."

Depression.

"When did you go to diabetes counseling?" he asks us.

"We didn't," I confess. "The clinic's first available appointment isn't until next Thursday."

"HMOs," our doctor grunts in dismay.

"So, the diet isn't working?" Francesca asks bravely.

"It's hard to know since you haven't had the benefit of professional guidance. You're doing your best, but it looks like you could still end up on insulin."

Insulin. That word again.

Francesca sighs deeply. "What are we facing?"

"The primary risk is high baby weight. People often say it's great to have a big baby, but that's not true. Large babies are more likely to have abnormalities. Also, unmanaged gestational diabetes can cause the fetus to fail." Our doctor speaks slowly and plainly. I appreciate his candor. "The good news is many women who successfully manage their condition deliver healthy babies."

Francesca clutches my hand.

"I'm sorry you have to wait so long to see a dietician," he adds. "You can thank your insurance company for that."

"This is Perry," I answer in my best business voice. I am working in my Home Office. Ten years ago it would have been called The Den.

"It's me," Francesca's voice is almost inaudible.

"Are you okay?"

"I fired Dr. Shell and got a Wednesday appointment with another specialist," her voice wavers. "I just cried in front of my boss."

A sharp, synthesized ring dissects her voice. "Gotta go, depot's on the other line."

"Call me back after you finish," I offer.

"Can't. I'm late for a meeting."

The line falls silent.

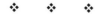

"You're not going to die?" Francesca's words awaken me from a dream. "Promise me you won't die." Her forehead creases with fear.

"I promise."

"Everything's so scary. We can die at any moment. Anywhere. Anytime."

"I know."

"It's horrible."

Francesca grabs Mister Fluffy for courage. For the first time, so do I.

"You're going to pull through this," assures our downy counselor.

I ponder my sudden, total surrender to Mister Fluffy. Intellectually, I know my impulsive, public embrace should cause me great embarrassment. But, it does not. Instead, the hug brings me relief and security. Without apology, I squeeze tighter.

"Don't worry," whispers Mister Fluffy. "No one will ever know."

❖   ❖   ❖

"Change in plans," Francesca speaks rapidly, her words accelerated by the entertainment industry's breakneck environment. "Dr. Shell's replacement just went out-of-network."

"What's that mean?" With one hand on the wheel and the other clutching my cell phone, I merge into five lanes of speeding traffic.

"It means our insurance company won't let us use him."

A BMW X5 moves within a foot of my bumper. I swerve left and offer its perfectly coifed driver my middle finger. "But it's been more than three weeks since your diagnosis."

"I found another guy," she continues. "He's in Tarzana. We'll see him next Tuesday."

"Tarzana?" I can't believe my ears. "That's an hour away."

A wall of traffic unexpectedly forms a few hundred yards ahead of me. I slow to a crawl, which soon deteriorates to a complete stop. To my right, the very same X5 that had been gunning for light-speed idles quietly.

Francesca's twelve-line phone roars to life. "Got to go. See you tonight."

Once again, hip-hop beats out the expectant father.

"Where is the park in office park?" I wonder aloud as we stand before the contractor-designed Tarzana Medical Associates office park. There are no swings, sandboxes or children. Lifeless, boxy buildings reign over acres of generic landscaping and asphalt. The only features remotely related to "park" are the parking spaces surrounding the concrete and glass complex.

I hold open a heavy steel door for Francesca. We navigate our way through a maze of narrow hallways, searching for suite 208. Two lefts and a right deliver us to the office. Its lobby feels oddly buoyant. Original prints hang from the wall. Interesting magazines boast unexpectedly current dates. A radiant bouquet adorns a reception counter and its frosted green glass window.

"Hi!" A jovial Indian woman slides open the glass. "You must be Francesca."

"Yes…" Francesca wonders why the receptionist is acting so friendly.

"Sorry to make you do this," the woman apologizes. "But you need to fill out these forms. Once you're done," she flashes a smile, "the doctor will be right with you."

Francesca embarks on a familiar journey through insurance claim documents, questionnaires and legal liability agreements. I brace myself for an insulting, endless wait. Within minutes of completing the required forms, the receptionist leads us to an exam room. I assume she is employing the old waiting room bait-and-switch tactic: create the impression of punctual service by shuttling patients from one holding area to another. I figure we will wait at least twenty minutes before we reach the real exam room.

"Hello," a youthful nurse greets us instantly. Her genuine glee chips away at my increasingly cynical view of healthcare. "Let's take a look at your baby."

A sonogram probe of Francesca's abdomen telegraphs vivid images to a wall monitor. Feet, toes, and a developing spine flash across the screen.

"Is the stomach size okay?" I ask. If the stomach is larger than the head, our baby is developing improperly.

"The proportions look perfect," reports the nurse.

Francesca takes my hand. "He's alright," she laughs.

"There's his brain." The nurse points a cursor at the baby's head. "And, that's his face."

Two closed eyes. A nose. A mouth. A mouth with lips like mine. A mouth sucking on an outstretched thumb.

Just as the sonogram ends, a tall, lanky man pops into the room. "Sorry to keep you waiting, I'm Doctor Ramsey." He shakes Francesca's hand. "Looks like you haven't gotten a chance to self-test your glucose levels."

"We've been trying to get equipment for weeks," I explain.

"Let's take care of that right now."

The doctor ferries us back the reception area and offers us a bright red box containing a Bayer Glucometer. Holding it in my arms brings both relief and unease. Relief for finding it. Unease for what it may tell us.

Gridlock on the 101 freeway. Only thirty minutes remain until show time. A quick survey of my backpack reveals I've forgotten to bring a potato. Without a potato, Act Two's restaurant scene is impossible. My only stage direction for the seven-minute sojourn is, "Pick at baked potato." To make matters worse, the woman playing my mother specifically asks me, "Why aren't you eating your potato?" and, in another moment, tells me to, "Eat your potato before it gets cold." If I were performing on Broadway, a stagehand would be responsible for the vegetable. But this is not Broadway. This is experimental, downtown Los Angeles theater. I must find a potato.

I check into a Kentucky Fried Chicken, otherwise known as KFC ever since the word "fried" became as taboo as plastic shopping bags.

"One baked potato, please," I request.

"We have mashed potatoes," replies a tattooed cashier. "No baked."

I speed down Sunset Boulevard and scan storefronts for another possible baked potato source: Taco Bell. Starbucks. McDonalds. Starbucks. 7-11. Starbucks. Winchell's. Starbucks.

A large fluorescent sign heralds Astro, a fifties diner.

I rush inside. "I need a baked potato."

"With or without sour cream?" asks the pink-haired hostess.

Thank God for Astro.

Glucometer Elite XL.

Francesca and I sit cross-legged at our living room coffee table.

Always wash and dry your hands before each test. Insert the test strip into the top of the Elite XL. Lance your finger and place blood on the test strip circle. A countdown meter will count down thirty seconds once there is enough blood on the test strip. Discard the lancet in its protective plastic cover.

Francesca inserts a needle into a spring-loaded, gray plastic lancer and slides a narrow plastic test strip into the glucometer.

"F-5," blinks the instrument's display panel.

"What's F-5 mean?" I ask.

"It means we're using the right kind of test strip." My wife cocks the lancer and places it against her right index finger. A curt "click" signals the lancet's penetration of skin. A blood drop oozes from the finger. Francesca spreads the crimson fluid on the test strip. The glucometer beeps. A count down clock appears on its display. *Twenty-Nine.* We hope for a good reading. *Sixteen.* We have no idea what good reading looks like. *Four.*

"One hundred thirty-two," flashes the glucometer.

"You got a one hundred thirty-two." I say.

"Yes," confirms Francesca. "I got a one hundred thirty-two."

We have no idea whether to laugh or cry.

"Welcome to the first night of the Beginning Parenthood class. We're going to talk about taking the baby's temperature, giving sponge baths and identifying signs of infection or sickness." Our instructor Barbara wipes clean an expansive dry-erase board. Her frosted blond hair cascades over a bulky, purple sweater.

Francesca and I sit among nineteen other couples, all of us expectant parents. One woman sports a crisp red business suit and impossibly perfect make-up.

"Isn't she a newscaster?" whispers someone.

Barbara embarks on a well-rehearsed routine. After distributing stapled handouts, glossy pamphlets and plastic babies, she opens with the first stunner of the evening.

"Don't ever use baby powder," she says. "Your infant can inhale it and develop respiratory problems." The class can't believe its ears. Barbara revels in our universal shock. She moves to the head of the class and takes center stage. She scans the room and launches the next salvo. "How many of you have chosen a pediatrician?"

Our embarrassed smiles betray the truth, no one has even thought about pediatricians. We can't believe our blatant stupidity.

"How many of you know what healthy baby poopy looks like?"

Spouses helplessly look to each other for a clue. None of us has any idea what a healthy poopy looks like.

"How many of you know how to give a proper sponge bath?" Our feet nervously tap the beige linoleum floor beneath us.

"It's alright," smiles the omniscient Barbara, "you're not alone."

We scan each other's faces to see if we've all reached the same horrible conclusion. We have. None of us knows the first thing about parenting. Put us in a room with a helpless newborn and the odds of its survival are worse than nil. Hand us a diaper and we'll put it on backwards. Tell us to prepare formula, and we'll concoct a mathematical equation.

"Cloth or disposable diapers?" Our instructor continues her studied performance.

"We're going to use cloth diapers," replies a smug-looking, thirty-something woman. Her face beams with confidence.

"Why?" Barbara welcomes the challenge.

"They're better for the environment," the woman replies smartly. Her round-shouldered husband nods weakly in approval. I know these people. Wealthy, pseudo-liberals who use politically correct euphemisms to disguise their hatred for just about everything. I can't resist.

"They use all sorts of harsh chemicals to clean cloth diapers," I report. "The chemicals end up in the Santa Monica Bay and poison dolphins."

Not a single dolphin lives in the Santa Monica Bay, but no politically correct person ever wants to be associated with killing Flipper. The woman turns white. I pegged her. She clutches her Lexus key-chain and recalls her recent one hundred-dollar donation to the Save Santa Monica Bay fund.

"He's right," chimes in our instructor. The death knell. "Cloth diapers are cleaned seven times in powerful bleaches and ammonia. All those chemicals go right down the drain into the ocean."

Francesca kicks my shin.

"Of course," continues Barbara, "disposable diapers aren't so great either." Politically correct, Lexus woman grins at me devilishly. "Even the newest disposable diapers will take five hundred years to decompose."

The dolphin-killer and I stare each other down until we realize our battle is doomed to a draw. Dead dolphins or landfills. You decide.

"Did you get an appointment with a dietician?" I have actually managed to catch Francesca between meetings. A miracle.

"None of the people Doctor Ramsey recommended are in-network." Only a pinhead HMO bureaucrat could have ever coined the term *in-network*.

"Well, then, who is?" I ask.

"Our insurance company is faxing me a list."

"You want me to make some calls?"

"No, I've got it handled."

"You're sure?" My voice betrays panic.

"Yes. I've got it covered. I will get an appointment."

"Promise?" I wonder if Francesca's condition will ever get the complete medical attention it deserves.

"Perry," Francesca's voice softens, "I promise. I'll get an appointment this week."

I feel remarkably powerless. I can't control Francesca's glucose level. I don't have the knowledge to devise her proper diet. I can't protect Enrico from diabetes. All I can do is wait. All I can do is hope. All I can do is pray.

"I'm so overwhelmed." Francesca never utters the word overwhelmed. She is Hollywood's Wonder Woman, the definition of unstoppable.

"I don't know if I can handle it," she sounds afraid. "The MC Pimpster advances have the wrong sticker."

"Francesca…"

"What?" She puts me on speakerphone.

"You're panicking about a CD called MC Pimpster."

"And?" She's too far gone.

I try another tact. "How about coming home early?" In the music industry that means before midnight.

"No. This has to be resolved." Francesca's office stereo blasts in the background. *In da buff. Get on da floor. Your face in the pillow. My woody wants more.*

"I got an appointment with a dietician." Dietician clashes with *woody*. Another one of Francesca's phones screams to life. "That's the printer. Gotta go."

My wife vanishes, her voice replaced by a dial tone.

Barbara, the Beginning Parenthood instructor, ferries us to the fourth stop on our hospital tour. "This is the LDR. The Labor and Delivery Room."

Our eyes move from a wall of tinted windows to a pale green metal bed. At the foot of the bed, a steel bar arches from one edge to the other. No one can take their eyes off the gleaming silver rod. It stirs thoughts of medieval times and the Spanish Inquisition.

"Pack socks in your hospital bag," advises Barbara, "the floor can get cold."

A hulking, metal-and-rivets, monster movie contraption lurks in a corner. Our instructor approaches it with a "Want to know what this is?" look on her face.

"This," she reveals, "is where they put your baby right after birth. It has a heat lamp to keep your newborn warm. Over there is the shower and a bathroom."

"What's the arched bar for?" one of the expectant mothers finally asks. Everyone prepares for the answer.

"That..." Barbara saunters over to the shimmering metal device. "...is the Squat Bar. Some women find it helps during labor."

The women turn pale. So do the men.

"It's a good idea to bring music," continues Barbara, oblivious to the unmistakable panic spreading through the room. "And, guys, don't forget food, you could be in this room for twenty-four hours."

Francesca and I grab each other. The joyous birthing fantasy perpetuated by pregnancy books has abruptly devolved into a hideous, primitive rite. Suddenly labor seems imminent and scary.

"Let's go to the nursery!" Barbara cheerfully bounds out of the room. Her class remains behind, paralyzed by the Squat Bar.

Francesca and I sit side by side, our legs tucked underneath the coffee table. The four-times-a-day ritual continues: engage lancet, puncture skin, spread blood on test strip, watch glucometer count down thirty seconds. We hope for a good reading—anything less than one hundred twenty and more than sixty. The seconds slowly descend.

"One hundred twenty-six," beeps Mr. Glucometer.

A squirrel scampers across our shingled roof. His footfalls and the monitor's chirps create an odd children's marching song. The pitter-patter of paws accelerates as the squirrel anticipates a bountiful supply of delicious acorns stashed in a nearby oak tree.

"It's less than one hundred thirty-two," Francesca observes hopefully.

"It's more than one hundred twenty," I reply bleakly.

"I guess that muffin killed me."

"What muffin?" I inquire.

No response.

"What muffin?" I repeat.

"I can't fucking believe it." I pace a tight circle in the kitchen. "How long is this going to last? I've been trying to get out of my contract for three months. Why is he keeping me? We're not making any money. What did I do to him?" I grab a handful of raw farfalle pasta, jam it into my mouth, and grind through the rigid bow ties one by one. "He's got a hundred other clients who make him money. I've just got me. I assume all the risk, and he cashes the checks."

"Be patient. You're almost free." Francesca helps herself to one-half cup of plain yogurt, the closest she can get to a milkshake without incurring the glucometer's wrath.

"It's this endless slow leak." I swallow the last bow tie and greedily seek out more comfort food. My eyes settle on an unopened box of Triscuits. "Every time I walk in there, he's just as busy as usual. Like it's a regular day while my career goes down the drain."

"You're going through a transition." Francesca tries to enjoy her bland meal.

"No argument there," I bark. "A transition from working actor to unemployed dad."

Classroom →. A blue rectangular placard guides us down an empty hallway.

We arrive at an unoccupied reception desk.

Classroom ←.

A passageway.

Classroom →.

A corridor awash in harsh fluorescent light.

Classroom ←.

Another hallway.

I'm beginning to think we've unwittingly stumbled upon Daedalus' labyrinth. Soon we'll be hopelessly lost, doomed to die under the hooves of a disgruntled Minotaur.

A grinning face from my past offers unexpected hope. A man in Ray-Ban sunglasses. A highway patrolman. A *ChiP.* Erik Estrada walks arm and arm with his beaming, pregnant wife.

"Excuse me..." I think of the innumerable hours spent watching Erik chase unmarked white Econoline vans down the 405 freeway.

"Looking for the Lamaze room?" he offers.

"Yes." *I'm talking to Officer Poncherello!*

"Down that hallway, take a left and then another right."

"Thanks."

"It's a great class." He flashes his trademark grin.

We watch Erik escort his wife down the corridor and disappear around a corner.

A blaring alarm clock tears me from a deep, restful sleep. Dull colors and gray spots flash before me as my eyes struggle to focus. I roll onto my stomach and stare at the hardwood floor. As my vision returns to its normal, substandard state, I notice a wisp of pink fabric peeking out from underneath the bed.

"Mister Fluffy?" I exclaim in disbelief.

"I told you the honeymoon would end." His words are barely audible.

"How long have you been down there?"

"Two weeks."

"Are you okay?"

"I'm fine."

"You sure?"

"No."

Mr. Fluffy slides back into his cave and takes his place among forgotten slippers and dust balls.

Doctor Braintree asks for the past week's glucose readings. Francesca obediently reports the results, which are carefully recorded in a battered spiral notebook: "Eighty-five. One hundred three. One hundred nine. One hundred fifty—"

"—What happened there?"

"Pizza happened there."

"Keep going."

"Ninety-four. Ninety-eight. One hundred eight. One hundred thirty."

Doctor Braintree grimaces.

"Pasta in tomato sauce," she explains.

"Half a cup?"

Francesca comes clean: "Two cups."

Doctor Braintree crosses his arms. "Go on," he exhales.

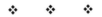

"He didn't say anything about insulin."

"No."

"That's good."

"I think so."

"He would have said something if it wasn't good."

"Right."

"Well then, that's good."

Francesca sleeps soundly while I stare at the ceiling, paralyzed by a single thought: *I've had no sex for two months.* I maneuver onto my left side and ponder the clock radio. New, more disturbing thoughts spawn from the first one: *We probably won't have sex until the baby's born. That's another month and a half.* I turn to talk radio for a much-needed diversion. The attempt fails. Conspiracy theories and alien hybridization are no match for my starved libido. *Didn't the Beginning Parenthood instructor say something about no sex until three months after the baby is born?* My stomach twirls. Fear compels me to do the math: *Two months plus a month and a half plus three months. That equals six and a half months. Six and one half months of no sex.* I flip onto my back and stare, once again, at the ceiling. I consider my options: *DVD or Internet. DVD or Internet. DVD or Internet.*

Colorful bags and brightly wrapped boxes. Barking dogs run circles around laughing children. Adults mill about the backyard congratulating us on our impending birth.

Francesca and I unwrap Enrico's gifts. One by one, our baby registry comes to life. A mobile. A vibrating seat. A fold-up bath tub. Shirts. Jumpsuits. A Sound-Soother. Lotion. Blankets. A Gyminie.

I find myself hovering above it all, watching me open gifts for my son. I see our friends, my father, and my cousins. I see Francesca. I see a life I have somehow created. A life born out of chaos, bad choices, luck, will and perseverance.

Only moments ago my mother held my hand and walked me from first to second grade homeroom.

"I'm never going to be in first grade again, will I?" I asked my mother.

"No, Perry, you won't."

First grade. Second grade. High school. College.

Engagement. Marriage. Baby Shower. Birth.

"I'm never going to be in first grade again, will I?"

"No, Enrico, you won't."

My father stretches out on an Adirondack chair and delves into a Thomas Mann novel. Sarah, his wife, sips iced tea and explores the latest *New Yorker*. For a rare moment, they disengage from their chronic, fourteen-hour workdays and embrace backyard leisure.

I carry a sack of presents from the garage through the patio and into Enrico's room. Francesca lies on the guest bed, her face pale.

"Enrico's not moving," she says.

"What?" Through an open window, I can see my father slowly drift off to sleep.

"He's not kicking. I don't feel him."

"Since when?"

"This morning."

"Before the baby shower?"

121

"Yes."

"Why didn't you say something?" Panic. "Why didn't you tell me?"

"Because," she groans, "I don't know."

"Let's do a kick count." I wrap my arms around Francesca's abdomen and wait for a reassuring thud. "The baby is supposed to kick ten times an hour."

"Do you feel anything?"

"No. Not yet." My hands sweep back and forth in search of a tap. The fingers strain. Ten minutes past two.

"There." My left pinky senses a minor vibration. "I think I felt something."

"Was it a kick?"

"I'm not sure."

Twenty-five minutes past two.

"We should call Doctor Braintree." I dart from the bed. "That's the thing to do."

"We don't need to bother him," protests Francesca.

I consider her objection for a moment and then reject it. An answering service informs me that Doctor Braintree is on his way to Hawaii for a well-earned vacation. In the interim another physician will treat his patients.

"Doctor Newfeld?"

"Yes?"

"We're first-time parents. We could just be over-reacting."

"Go on." The doctor's kind voice mixes a native French accent with an acquired California lilt.

"My wife has gestational diabetes, and our baby isn't moving much today. Usually he's very active. I'm wondering what we should do."

"Go to the hospital. Go right now."

"Right now?"

"Right now."

"Dad? Sarah?" I call out into the garden.

"Yes?" My father awakens from a light sleep.

"We're going to the hospital," I casually announce.

"Is everything alright?" Sarah peers out over *The Talk of the Town.*

"Everything's fine," is my placid reply. "We just noticed some slower fetal movement and since we're dealing with gestational diabetes, it's better to be safe than sorry."

"When will you be back?" My dad struggles to remain calm about the sudden turn of events.

"Two hours tops." I emphasize the word "tops" as if to imply our unexpected trip merits nothing more than a "Drive safely" in response.

"Drive safely," shouts Sarah.

We find ourselves back in the same labor and delivery room we visited two weeks ago, the one with the infamous squat bar. Everything looks the same except Francesca is lying on the metal bed, wrapped in monitoring devices. A strand of wires spans from Francesca's midsection to a rack of equipment composed of flashing lights, switches and a small television screen. Bright yellow numbers flicker across the monitor. One hundred forty-five. One hundred sixty-three. Francesca coughs violently. Each percussive hack opens her mouth wide, sends her tongue skyward and batters the lemon-color numbers down to one hundred ten.

"What do the numbers mean?" I ask a nurse.

"They track your baby's heartbeat which, twice every twenty minutes, should accelerate above normal levels."

A paper strip emerges from another section of the equipment. It passes underneath a quivering ink pen and cascades into a metal tray. The nurse tears off a section of the wavering, graphic data and jots notes on a manila file folder.

"How's Enrico doing?" I ask, hoping for a squiggly line translation.

"I see one acceleration." The nurse stands beside Francesca and offers her a glass of water. "When was the last time you ate?"

"About five hours ago." Francesca slurps down the liquid. "I had half a bagel and a mini muffin."

"That's all?" I ask in disbelief.

The nurse smiles momentarily and then returns her face to a professional, neutral countenance. "How about a turkey sandwich?"

"Okay," says Francesca, her eyes fixed on Enrico's heart rate.

"We'll take a glucose test before you eat." The nurse ventures down the hall in search of turkey.

"Can I have some more water?" Francesca asks in her sick voice. The consonants drip from her lips.

An orderly returns with a turkey on toasted rye. Francesca chews slowly, each swallow labored.

"Good girl," I congratulate my patient for finishing half of the sandwich.

Our nurse reappears twenty minutes after lunch and examines the paper strip's mysterious shivering line.

"There we go!" she exclaims.

"Two accelerations?" I ask.

"Four."

Thank God, I say to myself.

"Thank God," Francesca says aloud.

"You need rest." I notice our nurse's name tag for the first time. Joan White, R.N. continues, "You must eat regular, consistent meals."

Francesca promises to get more sleep. Francesca promises to eat. In this moment I can feel her finally surrender to pregnancy.

Hand in hand, Francesca and I walk down a long corridor lined with windows on the right and thick glass on the left. Something on the left stops us. Behind a thick translucent pane, a newborn stares out from a plastic crib. Her tiny arms and legs extend. We're frozen. Transfixed. The baby's right hand reaches into the air. Her eyes blink open and shut. She kicks. She screams.

Eight weeks and counting. Eight weeks and counting.

The sweet smells of garlic, onions and broiled fish waft through the house. My father and Sarah shuttle from stove to sink to refrigerator and back, preparing salmon steaks, vegetables, potatoes and exotic appetizers. Concern coats my father's face.

"The baby's alright," I say. "Francesca just needs some rest."

My father's face softens. His tense, upraised shoulders relax.

"We're making dinner," Sarah explains, as if she could be doing anything else with the pots and pans. "Are you hungry?"

"Yes." Francesca eyes me. "Very."

"This is from 1944." My father hands me a faded black and white photo. Twenty proud people wearing suits and dresses stare back at me. "This was taken during your great-grandparents' fiftieth wedding anniversary."

"Guess who that is!" chimes in Sarah.

A small boy in a gray suit.

"Dad?" I guess.

"That's right," she confirms.

I examine the photographed faces one by one and recognize only four: my grandfather, grandmother, uncle and father. All the other mouths, eyes and bodies are unknown.

A thought: I would not exist if they had not existed.

Anonymous faces, my flesh and blood.

"What was my great-grandfather's name?" I ask.

"Harold. And your great-grandmother was Etta."

I examine my ancestors' traits closely, searching for a hint of my face and body.

"Where were they born?"

"Somewhere in Eastern Europe." My father does not know.

I imagine myself walking through a Polish village at the turn of the century and greeting a young man as I would any stranger, a tip of the hat. I continue down a cobblestone walkway, unaware I have just met my great-great-grandfather.

I wonder if a cousin died in the Holocaust. I wonder if a great uncle was an inventor or a soldier. I wonder if a distant relative painted during the Renaissance. I will never know. I live in the forever present. Sit-coms, movies, and traffic are my personal history.

"Where was my great-great-grandmother born?" asks Enrico.

"I don't know."

"When did she come to America?"

"I don't know."

A guttural cough drags me from a deep sleep. Francesca convulses and twists. Labored deep breaths signal congestion and thick phlegm.

"You need a drink." I embark on a dizzy journey to the refrigerator and its Brita water pitcher.

"I'm alright," calls out Joan of Arc. Another explosive hack rebounds off the walls and ceilings.

Francesca sputters between gulps of water. Gradually the breathing eases. The face relaxes.

"I'm sick," she says.

"Yes," I confirm, "you're sick."

Francesca sucks on a thermometer originally intended for Enrico.

"Ninety-nine and a half," I report. "That's better."

"Can you pull the comforter up over me?" My wife's unguarded face betrays her absolute exhaustion.

I pull the duvet up to her neck, tuck the bed sheets and puff the pillows. Francesca's body contorts sharply. The recurring, ragged hack rumbles, once again, from her bronchioles, through her esophagus and into the room. Another one follows. And another. Francesca clutches her chest.

A sugar-free Ricola soothes the ravaged throat.

"This is Francesca Manarola. I will out of the office all day Monday. I will be checking my voicemail. If this is a production emergency, dial 555-1200."

"This is Francesca Manarola. I will out of the office all day Tuesday. I will be checking my voicemail. If this is a production emergency, dial 555-1200."

"This is Francesca Manarola. I will out of the office all day Wednesday. I will be checking my voicemail. If this is a production emergency, dial 555-1200."

"I'm home." My arms overflow with groceries.
"Hi." Francesca waves from the kitchen.
"She walks."
"I walk."
Francesca returns to the world of the living.

Childlike cartoons, tacked to the wall, illustrate an expectant mother's journey through delivery. Bold-faced captions define each stage:

Early Labor. A calm face.
Active Labor. A concerned face.
Transitional Labor. A grimacing face.
Pushing. A spent face.

I notice the conspicuous absence of a smiling face. So do the pregnant women.

"Pain Management and Medication," exclaims this evening's pamphlet.

Fifteen couples sit on thin foam exercise mats. Some women massage their abdomens while others struggle to stay awake. Some men rub their wives' shoulders while others struggle to stay awake.

Tonight's instructor, Jennifer, sports a flowered print dress and a smart wool sweater. New Age and serenity ooze from her espadrilles. She inhales deeply, "It's a cleansing breath followed by short, shallow breaths."

Jennifer floats among us, observing the women's breathing technique, the key to surviving transitional labor. Each mother-to-be clutches an ice cube, which simulates the constant pain of rapid contractions. Droplets of frosty water drip from their palms.

"And the contraction begins." Jennifer makes a note of the time. Her perpetually cheery disposition buoys the women's hopes for a tolerable birth. Her calming tones encourage the mothers to envision a journey ending in happiness rather than irrevocable physical trauma.

Francesca and I face each other, my legs crossed, hers outstretched.

As a birthing-coach-in-training, it is my responsibility to guide my wife through the process. "Take your cleansing breath," I say.

Francesca inhales. The remnants of her cold bar her from capturing a full breath.

"Twenty seconds." Jennifer marks the time. Francesca maintains a firm grip on the ice cube. Her breaths grow shallow. Her face turns anxious. Her body becomes rigid. The sudden change in temperament seems unbelievable and melodramatic. I hide my doubt behind a smile.

"The ice cube's cold," Francesca snaps angrily. The clairvoyant.

"Hold on." I pretend not to notice her ire. "You can do it, I know you can."

"The contraction is peaking." Jennifer signals the forty-five second mark.

"Look into my eyes," I command. Our eyes lock. "Three shallow breaths. Three shallow breaths." I raise my right hand and signal each breath with an extended finger.

"Heee. Heee. Heee," exhales Francesca.

I make a fist, the symbol for a gradual, full inhalation. Francesca obediently follows my direction. A relaxed breath wipes away the ice-cube-induced pain.

"The contraction is leveling off," announces Jennifer.

Francesca exhales easily. A smile washes over both our faces.

"The breathing works!" Francesca spurts in amazement.

"And the contraction is over," Jennifer ends the exercise.

The room is abuzz. Couples excitedly share their experiences with each other. Joy spreads around the workout mats. *The breathing works! The breathing works!* Hope lives at tonight's Lamaze class.

Plastic infant mannequins. *A is for airway. B is for breathing. C is for circulation.* Baby CPR class.

Two women, a couple, sit together at one end of a faux wood collapsible table. Francesca and I sit at the other end, shifting endlessly in rigid, folding metal chairs. A graying father and a brunette mom tend to their five-month-old boy. A solo mother explores the contents of her blue vinyl handbag. A man with a deformed right arm sits next to his turtleneck wife.

"The baby is unconscious. Her airway is blocked." Our instructor, Barbara, leads us through an emergency scenario. "What do you do?"

I rest a plastic infant on my left arm, stomach down. With the heel of my right hand, I hit her upper back five times. I turn over the baby, making sure to support the neck, find the center point between her breasts, measure one finger down, and, with two vertical fingers, apply five thrusts.

"She's still unconscious," warns Barbara.

I insert a thumb into the baby's mouth and check for obstructions. I tilt her head back until it is parallel with the ceiling, place my mouth over her nose and mouth, and push air into her lungs.

"She's not breathing." Another troubling update from Barbara.

Once again, I lay the baby on my left arm, stomach down. I strike her back five times, turn her over and thrust two fingers against the chest area.

"She gasps for air!" Barbara's play-by-play continues. "What's this mean?"

"The airway is clear?" A cautious suggestion from the graying father.

"That's right. You've got A. Now what?"

"Check for breathing and circulation," recommends Francesca.

"Correct. Everyone check B and C."

My right hand rests on the baby's left armpit and searches for a heartbeat.

"There's a pulse," reports Barbara, right on cue. "But now the baby isn't breathing."

"Rescue breathing," I spout.

"That's right." Our instructor beams with pride.

"And two and three," I count aloud as I blow more air into the plastic body.

"You're gonna do twenty cycles of this," directs Barbara.

I run through twenty cycles.

My plastic daughter takes a sudden turn for the worst. Barbara delivers the bad news, "The circulation stops."

"Full CPR," commands Perry Herman, MD.

Two fingers position themselves just below the baby's breast line. I count to five, pressing firmly against the baby's chest with each audible.

"Do your A-B-C check."

Doctor Herman administers the check.

"She's breathing," announces Barbara. "Circulation is back. The airway is clear. You just saved your baby."

Shoulders relax. Focus widens.

"Good job!" Barbara congratulates her new flock of emergency medical technicians.

"Everything's going to be alright," I assure my plastic baby, "Daddy's right here."

A tube of textured rubber expands, then contracts. Lips wrap tightly around a cold metal valve. A hearty exhalation transforms the deformed material into a rigid ring. Clumsy fingers struggle to seal the valve before precious air is lost. The red cushion's skin loosens ever so slightly.

"Ready." I solemnly place the donut on a nearby dining chair.

Francesca examines the object's irregular, elastic surface. Certain of its stability, she edges lower until her full weight rests on the cherry-colored lifesaver.

"Ah," she exhales. "I can sit again."

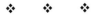

The stone covered interior courtyard teams with laughing, vibrant office workers. Thick white frosting encases a festive carrot cake. Blue icing weaves across the white expanse to spell *Enrico*. Bright gift-wrapped boxes blanket a long buffet table. My mother, Francesca and I stare in disbelief. It appears my wife's coworkers have purchased everything on our registry. Francesca's boss, Phil, embraces her. His eyes beam with warmth. He, too, will soon be a father.

"Open your gifts!" shouts someone.

We oblige and tear through packing tape and colorful paper. Enrico's spoils peek out from inside their cardboard containers:

The Peg-Perego Prima Pappa. The Range Rover of highchairs.

The Peg-Perego Venezia. The BMW of strollers.

The Graco Pack N' Play. The Cadillac of portable playpens.

With the last gift opened, a horde descends upon the cake leaving only an "O" on its once pristine shell. Soon the fear of unread, urgent e-mails and unheard, emergency voicemails send the revelers back to their flashing phones and whirring computers. The courtyard falls silent.

Phil and I guide a mailroom dolly filled with presents into an awaiting elevator.

"Wow," I say as we descend to the garage. "We never expected so much."

"Are you kidding?" laughs Phil.

I force the last box into the Maxima's passenger compartment and shut a rear door just before another carton falls back out onto the garage floor. I consider the car's unusual state. It looks like a mobile baby superstore. Infant gear fills every nook and cranny of the rolling glass and steel showroom. The once familiar cloth bucket seats have vanished, leaving me with a serious puzzle to solve: Where will we sit?

"How about here, above the changing table?" I hold a newly assembled IKEA LUND shelf up against a wall.

"Too dangerous!" My mother submarines the idea.

"It could fall on the baby," implores Jan, my mother's partner.

"What about here?" I move the shelf left.

"Don't have anything above the table," urges Jan.

"How about on the floor?" my mother suggests. "Below the window."

"It would be too hard to reach," pipes in Francesca. She wants the shelf placed exactly where I'm holding it.

"Here's a thought." I rest the LUND on the table. Due to its unusual Swedish design, it looks both fashionable and sturdy. The women of my life consider the unexpected proposal.

"Good," approves Mom.

"Safer," applauds Jan.

"Convenient," adds Francesca.

We admire Enrico's nursery: Wooden crib, Fischer Price Sound Shaper, Sony baby monitor, John Lennon Imagine elephant, teddy bear mobile, nightlight, Winnie the Pooh blanket, changing table, LUND shelves, baby-wipe warmer, Evenflo humidifier, and yellow walls.

"This room is ready for a baby," observes Jan. She's right. It is.

I unpack my childhood library and carefully arrange its contents on a low, wooden bookcase. The musty, reassuring scent of aged paper reminds me of story time with my mother and father. Mike Mulligan, Ping and Ferdinand line up next to Curious George, the Little Prince and Policeman Small. Mr. Small, a smartly uniformed patrolman, calls out from his gray hardback book. Unsteady handwriting scrawled across the book's title page identifies its current owner: Perry. Immediately familiar drawings spring forth from the glossy pages: Policeman Small directing traffic with his portable stop sign, Policeman Small taking an accident report, Policeman Small waving "Hello" to the milkman.

Soon Enrico will know Policeman Small.

Soon Enrico will idolize Policeman Small's ability to keep the streets safe.

Soon Enrico will pass Policeman Small onto the next generation: His son. My grandchild.

A poorly orchestrated "Yankee Doodle Dandy" blurts from my cell phone, reminding me, once again, it's time to choose another ring setting.

"Hi," Francesca's voice strains with urgency.

"You sound terrible." I prepare for the worst.

"Doctor Braintree wants to know why I haven't had any non-stress tests."

"That's easy," I reply. "He hasn't done any."

"He thought Doctor Ramsey was doing them."

"Why would he think that?"

"I guess I dropped the ball," Francesca's voice fractures "I guess it was my responsibility."

"No," my neck stiffens, "it wasn't."

"He said it might be necessary to induce labor or do a cesarean," her words continue, oblivious to my answers. "After thirty-eight and a half weeks, all the baby does is gain weight."

"What is wrong with him? Why is he talking about a cesarean?" My whole body seizes with anger.

"I don't know," Francesca whispers. "I don't know."

"This is bullshit," I bark. "Total bullshit."

"I'm so sorry." Her apology shrinks to nothing, the *sorry* barely audible.

Francesca's deepening grief awakens me from my angered craze. I realize my wife needs compassion, not a barrage of furious questions and cuss words.

"You didn't do anything wrong," I assure her.

"I didn't hurt the baby?"

"No, Enrico is fine."

"Positive?" her voice wobbles.

"Completely."

"I'm so worried." The consonants and vowels dissolve into sobs and tears.

Doctor Braintree settles behind his aging desk and offers me a low-back chair. The wooden golden retriever eyes us both.

"We've been here three times," I struggle to contain my emotions. "There's been no testing. And today you made Francesca feel like it's all her fault."

Doctor Braintree offers me a striped spearmint candy. "I thought your other physician was doing them."

"Did Doctor Ramsey say he was?"

"I haven't spoken to him yet."

I am stunned by the revelation. "Francesca is *terrified* she's hurt the baby."

"I've never met Doctor Ramsey." The veteran practitioner rubs his creased forehead. "Your insurance company hasn't even given me his phone number." Doctor Braintree rests his elbows on a mound of paperwork. "I'm getting too old for this," he tells himself.

"What's this about a cesarean?" I continue, a bit less fire in my belly.

"I'm legally bound to inform you of all possible risks associated with gestational diabetes. I don't think Francesca will need one."

"Okay." All of his answers are reasonable.

I thank the doctor for his time, wondering if I've just shot the messenger, and step into chaos: Nurses shuttle between occupied examination rooms. An office manager battles a faceless insurance administrator: "So we're supposed to eat the fee?" she snaps incredulously into her phone. An assistant wanders about aimlessly. "Who needs these test results?" she asks no one in particular. Restless patients check and re-check their watches. "Why is he so behind?" they mutter to themselves.

I consider the nightmare facing our doctor: insurance plans that limit treatment options, HMOs barring referrals to lifelong colleagues, and swarms of attorneys, ready to sting.

I imagine a time in the not too distant future. A time without obstetricians. A time when attorneys and insurance administrators deliver all the babies.

"You have to feel this! Put your hand here!" Francesca places my right palm on her abdomen. A foot pushes out. A leg moves up and back. A hand taps against mine.

I introduce myself to Francesca's stomach, "Hi, Enrico. This is your dad."

The abdomen bulges under the pressure of an extended knee.

"Uhhh," moans Francesca.

"Enrico, how about less knee and more foot?"

The knee extends again. This time further.

Something tells me my son has a strong point of view. Something tells me he will be a handful. Something tells he will be more than I've ever imagined. I can't wait to meet him.

"I'm burning up." Sweat drips from Francesca's pores.

"Did you take Tylenol?"

"Yes." She buries her head under a pillow.

"Robitussin, too?"

"Yes."

Enrico's thermometer blinks "100.4." I recall something we learned in a Lamaze class: *If the pregnant mother's temperature remains at 100.4 for more than six hours, she must go to the hospital. No ifs, ands or buts.*

Two in the morning. Francesca climbs back into bed.

"99.8," she reports.

"That's good," I say from a dream.

Days tumble towards me. The moment approaches. "Enrico." Coming to a hospital near you.

I twist the tuning knob on my handheld, ten-band world radio, hoping to intercept the BBC and its familiar station identification: the chimes of Big Ben followed by "This is London," spoken in an aristocratic British dialect.

Francesca rocks back and forth, trying to build enough momentum to sit upright in our Shabby Chic bed.

"This is so humiliating," she sighs.

I crawl behind Francesca and apply increasing pressure to her lower back until our combined efforts launch her into a seated position. She extends her legs downward and, in a less than graceful maneuver, slides off the mattress and crashes to the floor. My exhausted, full-term pregnant wife eyes the bathroom door.

"That's why you must beg God for mercy!" blurts a voice from the radio. Southern accent. Fire and brimstone. Definitely not London.

"Help," cries Francesca from the bathroom.

Acting as a human cantilever, I lift Francesca off the toilet and lead her back to the bedroom.

"I'm so ready to have this baby," she mutters as she stands before our unusually high bed frame. To her chagrin, her right leg cannot lift high enough to clear the mattress. Neither can her left.

"If you tell anyone about this, you're dead." Francesca grabs the sheets and, using them like a rope, pulls herself up onto the bed. She looks like a confused escaped convict trying to break back into prison.

"Maybe we should get a step stool," I suggest.

Francesca pulls the covers over her head and mutters angry gibberish into a pillowcase.

I spread a paper napkin across my khaki lap.

Elliot, a friend from my advertising days, shares stories about his four-month-old daughter, Jane. He tells me about her first laughs, her first cold and the time she spit up on his new suit. My mind drifts from the joyous yarns to an unfamiliar image hovering in a mirror just behind Elliot's head: a face. My face. Pimples line the left cheek. Red blotches populate the jaw and neck. Dark bags slump beneath bloodshot eyes. A worn-out father-to-be stares back at me.

"I look like shit," I say aloud.

"You do look a bit ragged, my friend," confirms Elliot.

"Francesca has been sick for days. She keeps waking up every two hours." Recalling the recent past drains me of all remaining energy; my shoulders sag under the weight of constant stress and sleep deprivation.

"Anything to drink?" asks a perky, chin-pierced waiter.

"Whatever you get," suggests Elliot, "make sure it's ninety-eight percent caffeine."

Heading his advice, I utter three simple words: "Diet Coke. Large."

"That's my man," cheers Elliot. "That's my man."

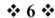

❖ 6 ❖

Dimas, the El Salvadoran painter from Lee Kim Interiors, applies a third coat of white to the foyer ceiling. The living room glistens, the previously dingy surfaces rejuvenated with red, forest green and mustard yellow.

I scan my Internet start page for news headlines: *Israel and PLO Set to Talk, Congress Gridlocked, Microsoft on the Rise.*

"If only I'd bought Microsoft five years ago," I mutter to myself. Memories of prior investment *What ifs?* rush forward. "If only I'd sold AOL four years ago. If only I'd bought—"

"—Perry?" Francesca calls from the opposite end of the house. "Come here!"

I follow her voice to a closed bathroom door. "Do you need some toilet paper?"

"No!" she whispers urgently.

The white wooden door swings open to reveal a frightened Francesca sitting on the toilet, her hands gripping the rim.

"It's like a waterfall." She points between her legs.

"Oh my God." The moment has arrived. "Your water broke!"

"It's just a big pee," snips Francesca.

I dart down the hallway. "We're going to the hospital."

"It's two weeks too soon."

I wheel a densely packed overnight bag towards the front door.

"My water hasn't broken," Francesca persists. "Call a nurse at the hospital. She'll tell you."

I scan our refrigerator door for Doctor Braintree's telephone number. My fingers dial the eleven digits quickly. Three piercing tones leap from the handset. "The number you have dialed has been disconnected," reports a dispassionate female voice. "Hang up and please try again." A second attempt connects me with the same soulless woman. I breathe deeply and dial the numbers as slowly as possible.

"Doctor Braintree's office, how can I help you?"

"This is Perry Herman. I need to speak to the doctor immediately."

"He's on vacation."

"Still?" I exclaim in disbelief.

"Would you like me to page Doctor Newfeld?"

"Yes!" I blurt. "Please."

Silence.

"Sir?"

"Uh-huh?"

"What's your phone number?"

"Uh," I struggle to recall the ten most familiar digits in my life. "Three-two-three...five-five-five...zero-eight...one...five."

"The doctor will call you right back."

Silence.

"Mr. Herman?"

"Yes?"

"You need to hang up. No one can call you back if you're still on the line."

Her logic is undeniable. I hang up.

Francesca remains firmly fixed to the toilet.

"It's alright, Perry," she assures me. "I'm just peeing a lot."

"Have you ever peed for ten minutes?"

Francesca struggles with the question.

"How about five?"

Francesca does the math.

"How about two?"

The equation does not compute.

The phone rings.

"My wife started peeing about ten minutes ago, and she hasn't stopped."

139

"Go to the hospital," orders Doctor Newfeld.

"Now?"

"Now."

"Well?" Francesca asks smartly.

"We're going to the hospital."

"But, I've got production meetings, a finance luncheon, a graphics—"

I rush past Dimas, the painter. "We're having a baby!"

Dimas applies another layer of bright mustard yellow paint. "Buona suerte," he cheers, "Buona suerta."

I stare intently at the dashboard, making sure not to exceed the speed limit.

Francesca barks commands into her cell phone, "Put the single on manufacturing hold until the mastering studio gets its act together." We're on our way to have a baby, and my wife is doing business. "No," she continues, "today doesn't work, but tomorrow morning is open. Let's make it ten."

"You're going to be booked," I warn.

"Todd, call Phil." Francesca scans her Palm Pilot. "Tell him I will be available tomorrow around two."

"Honey, you're not getting the picture." I guide the car into the hospital's Urgent Care driveway.

"Damn," she grumbles. "Eleven voicemail messages."

I haul the luggage out of the trunk and roll it around to the front. I tap the car key against Francesca's window. "Let's go!"

"Just a second!"

"No more calls."

"Last one!" The cell phone junky enters a flurry of digits. "This is Francesca Manarola," her words are calm and collected. "I will be out of the office today. Please direct all inquiries to Mary at extension four-five-six-seven."

"That's it," I shout.

"One more." Her fingers reach for the keypad.

"—Francesca!"

"What?"

"You're having a baby!"

An orderly hands me a clipboard packed with disclaimers, forms and waivers. "Mr. Manarola?"

"Actually, I'm Mr. Herman. My wife didn't take my last name. So I'm not Mr. Manarola. But, I am her husband. If that makes any sense." It doesn't.

A young South American nurse rolls a gleaming stainless steel wheelchair towards Francesca.

"I'm fine. I can walk." Francesca demonstrates her agility by trotting around the waiting room. "See? I'm not really in labor. My husband thinks my water broke. But, it hasn't."

"Hospital rules," replies the nurse kindly. "All women in labor must be taken upstairs in a wheelchair."

"But, you see, that's the whole thing. I'm not in labor."

The LDR. The labor, delivery and recovery room. Only moments ago we were here for Francesca's mini-muffin emergency. The hulking baby warmer greets us like an old friend. A stethoscope hangs from a shelf. The familiar monitors and wires await.

A short Indian nurse in pink scrubs scribbles remarks on a clipboard. "I'm Kamla," she says to the equipment.

"Nice to meet you," I reply warmly, remembering our Lamaze teacher's advice: *Always be nice to the nurses. They run the place.* "This is Francesca," I motion to my barely clothed wife, "and I'm Perry, her husband." *Her husband?* Who else would I be? I berate myself for making such a stupid remark.

"Are you allergic to any anesthesia or pain killers?" Kamla asks matter-of-factly.

"No," replies a barefoot Francesca. She struggles to secure a paper-thin white robe around her body. Two scrawny tie-strings offer the only dim hope of achieving her goal.

"Lie down." The nurse acts like a bored airline pilot, plodding through a pre-flight checklist for the thousandth time.

Francesca lies down. Kamla rolls a tall metal pole towards the bed. Transparent plastic bags dangle from the pole's outstretched arms. Stamped on one bag is an illegible word and, on the other, Dextrose.

"What are in the sacks?" I ask.

"Saline solution and Pitocin."

Pitocin, the dreaded drug our instructor Jennifer told us to avoid at all costs. "Doctors will try to give you Pitocin to accelerate your delivery," she had warned us. "But, trust me," she took a long, dramatic pause, "you can't imagine how much more painful your contractions will be."

"Is Doctor Newfeld available?" I ask gingerly.

"Why?" Not the reassuring response I expected.

"I want to talk about our options."

"*Options*?" I have offended our nurse.

"Well. Just that…" *Always be nice to the nurses. They run the place.* "…if we put Francesca on Pitocin now, her contractions will be much worse."

Kamla's face turns to stone. "Francesca isn't dilated," she replies curtly. "There's no sign of effacement. And, as far as contractions are concerned, she has none." *You do the math* say her narrowing eyes.

Francesca fires back, "Our Lamaze teacher told us to walk around. She said it stimulates contractions and dilation."

"You can't *walk around* after your water breaks." Kamla regards her dismissively. "If you did, you'd risk losing amniotic fluid which can cause serious fetal infections."

Francesca backpedals. "What if we wait a while?"

"For what?" The stark brevity of Kamla's answer robs of us of any immediately obvious reply. Kamla fills the sudden, awkward silence, "You can either start Petocin now, or sit around and add another eight hours to your labor." She pauses and then tosses out a curt: "It's your choice."

Francesca and I look to each other for another tactic, another way out of this unexpected turn of events. We can both feel our fully natural labor quickly transforming into a fully drug-induced medical procedure.

"Go ahead," surrenders Francesca.

Within seconds an intravenous tube runs from the Petocin bag down through a baby blue IVAC box and into a metal needle lodged in Francesca's bloodstream. My eyes fix on the blue box. A small screen displays the number 72.0 in gray liquid crystal digits. I rub Francesca's legs and offer her a supportive smile. She smiles stoically. A vindicated Kamla collects her belongings and marches out of our room.

The IVAC's tiny screen now displays 74.0. Somehow Kamla managed to increase the Pitocin dosage without my noticing. I wonder if Francesca is being punished for our insubordination.

"Take that!" I imagine our nurse growling to herself as she ratchets up the pain machine.

Francesca clicks away at a remote control hoping to find something other than soap operas and talk shows. Every program looks the same. A sorry-looking twenty-year-old Zenith flashes one defective, grainy picture after another. People with pink skin stand before orange clouds. I wonder why the ancient television doesn't come crashing down from the ceiling. Only a paltry metal wall bracket keeps gravity from taking its toll.

"Can I have some ice chips?" asks Francesca.

I grab a pitcher of frozen slivers and dole out a serving. "How about some music?" I suggest.

"Okay." Francesca wears the face of a frightened child.

"Francesca would feel better on her back," advises Kamla.

"Right." I jump, startled by our nurse's sudden, unannounced return.

"What did you say?" she demands.

"Right, as in yes or good idea." I wonder how she re-entered the room without making a sound.

Kamla eyes me suspiciously and edges towards Francesca. In one swift, unexpected motion, she pulls a bed sheet out from underneath my wife's swollen body. It rolls awkwardly from side to back.

"How's that?" quips the platoon leader.

"Much better!" Francesca works overtime to express her appreciation.

Kamla glances at her watch, does a quick calculation, and reaches for the Petocin dispenser.

"What are you doing?" I blurt.

"My job." The cold reply. 74.0 climbs to 74.5.

"Are you having a boy or girl?"

"A boy," I offer cautiously.

"I got married too early," Kamla confides. "Had a kid at twenty-one. Now I'm old."

I remain silent, confused by the sudden, intimate confession.

"If I could do it all over," she continues, "I wouldn't have married, and I certainly wouldn't have had a kid. I would have traveled."

"Travel is very rewarding," I reply neutrally.

"If you need anything, just push the call button." Kamla smiles wistfully, collects her papers, and disappears, once more, down the hallway.

An ear-piercing scream bores through a wall of the LDR. A young woman begs for mercy. "No! No!" she cries. "Please...No..."

Snippets of other muffled voices trickle into our room. "Relax...breathe...you must breathe..."

Kamla returns, clipboard in hand, stethoscope swinging from her neck.

"What's happening next door?" I ask.

Francesca sits up in bed; her hands grip the metal railing. "It sounds like someone is dying."

"No one is dying," replies Kamla offhandedly. "A fifteen-year-old girl is in labor. She's terrified."

A shriek rings out, "Pleeeeeeease!"

"Relax...Breathe..." Barely audible voices answer her call. "You've got to keep breathing..."

Kamla's jaw tenses. "She's all alone, except for her aunt and teenage boyfriend."

"I can't imagine," is all I can say.

"Labor is much more painful when the mother is afraid." Kamla records Francesca's vital signs.

"Where's my mother?" shouts the teenager. "Where's my mother?"

"You're much more prepared than she is," says Kamla warmly. "You've taken classes, and you've got a very good coach." And with that, the mercurial Kamla exits our room.

A ceaseless stream of paper flows from the bedside fetal monitor and cascades onto the gray-specked linoleum floor. The now familiar, continuous black wavering line travels up and down the paper's grid-covered skin. Along the narrow display panel, the glowing heart flashes on and off, and orange numbers race from 100 to 150 and back. I glance at an ancient wall clock, hoping to calculate the elapsed time. Three hours and ten minutes. I note the Petocin dispenser's current dosage rate: 76.0. Francesca groans in pain.

"You want some painkiller?" Kamla asks Francesca.

"Yes." Not the answer I expected. "Anything to take the edge off." *Anything to take the edge off?* In less than a few hours, my wife has transformed into a junkie, desperate for a fix. *Any fix.*

Kamla produces a syringe and within seconds injects soothing Demerol into Francesca's forearm. "You let me know if you want an epidural."

"Thanks," replies Francesca lustfully.

"How are you doing?" slips from my lips. I'm amazed by the stupidity of my question.

"How does it look like I'm doing?" growls Francesca. "And stop rubbing my leg, it's annoying."

I discover my right hand has been rubbing Francesca's left shin in an endless, unrelenting circular motion. A comforting massage has mutated into a perpetual Indian rope burn.

145

Kamla returns to evaluate the dilation status. "Two centimeters," she reports.

"Two?!" Francesca cries in disbelief.

"How about the contractions?" I inquire, hoping for a better answer.

"Still very far apart." The unwelcome truth.

"The drug isn't doing anything." Francesca rubs her eyes. "I need something else." A wave of panic crashes over her. "Something stronger."

I bolt for the nurses' station and find Kamla engaged in a leisurely conversation about nothing in particular.

"My wife needs more medication," I plead.

Kamla feigns a smile. "Be right there."

As I sprint back to the LDR, I realize this marks the first time I've scored drugs for my wife.

Kamla returns much after *Be right there*. "You want the epidural?" she snips.

"Yes!" is the urgent reply.

Our enigmatic nurse departs, promising fast relief.

I hold Francesca's hand and repeat the words of our Lamaze instructor. "Deep breaths. From the abdomen."

Francesca welcomes the opportunity to focus on respiration, praying it will help her forget the constant, stabbing back pains. With each exhalation, her stern expression gradually relaxes.

"I'm Doctor Bruge." The anesthesiologist rummages through his coat hoping to find something, possibly a business card or a pen. "Sit up so that your back is to me."

I offer my arm for support, but Francesca declines, preferring the assistance of her own muscles.

"Now," continues the physician, "hunch over and remain as still as possible."

"Still?" quips Francesca. "What if I'm having a contraction?"

"Just try not to move."

Francesca positions herself while Doctor Bruge prepares an absurdly long needle which, thankfully, is beyond his patient's peripheral vision. He carefully positions the syringe and presses firmly on its plastic plunger. Francesca sighs happily; only minutes separate her from serenity.

Wires and tubes spring from every side of Francesca's body: two in her left forearm, one draped on her leg, three spiraling out of her stomach and one, the epidural, protruding from her back. Machines and monitors bleep, click and gurgle. Beep, click and gurgle. Francesca looks like a science experiment, a creature borne from some crazed researcher's perverse dream. She has become a specimen tethered to a mattress Petri dish.

"How are you doing, Francesca?" An unfamiliar nurse whirls into the room.

"Where's Kamla?" I ask. Who cares? I think.

"Shift change. I'm Yvette."

Fate has blessed us with Kamla's polar opposite. Yvette is the picture of compassion and professionalism.

"I'm so glad you're here," I spout a bit too eagerly.

Yvette immediately gets down to business. "Girl?"

"Yes," gurgles Francesca.

"What are you doing on your back?"

"The other nurse told me I'd be more comfortable."

"Child, you're in the worst posture imaginable. It doesn't stimulate contractions and certainly isn't encouraging your baby to come on out." Yvette positions herself alongside the bed. "We're going to rotate your wife," she explains. "On a count of three, grab hold of her right side and push."

I await the count.

"One. Two. Three."

In one swift motion Francesca rolls onto her right side. The fetal monitor screams in protest. Yvette moves to the foot of the bed and examines Francesca's dilation. "Still two centimeters."

"I can't feel my legs." Francesca's voice sounds strained, as if her chest were collapsing under an immense weight. "I can't feel my arms."

"What do you mean?" I ask.

"Exactly what I said." Her breathing grows shallow.

Yvette presses a blunt probe into Francesca's left forearm. "Can you feel that?"

"No," is the winded reply.

Yvette slides the probe to the upper arm and presses again. "How about that?"

"Nothing."

"What's going on?" I sense something serious and unexpected.

"It's the epidural." Yvette whips around the bed and disengages the drug.

"What's the situation?" Doctor Bruge materializes, his face stern and fixed.

"She's T3," reports Yvette.

"T3?" His voice flutters ever so slightly.

"Chest constriction as well."

"Pulse-ox monitor." The anesthesiologist grabs a chair, positions it next to the bed, and sits down.

Yvette passes a long black wire to the doctor who attaches it to Francesca's index finger. Another region of the fetal monitor awakens and displays a mysterious 92%. Uneven respiration accompanies the new number. Francesca's upper chest rises and falls in quick, sharp spurts. Each gasp sends Enrico's heart rate spiraling downward. I am in an unreal dream.

"Ten milliliters of epinephrine," calls out the doctor. Yvette produces a syringe. Swift pressure to its plunger sends clear liquid speeding toward Francesca's already flooded bloodstream.

"What's happening?" I blurt.

"Oxygen," commands the doctor. A clear-plastic mask is secured over Francesca's mouth and nose.

"What's happening?" I repeat, this time louder.

The doctor pulls back and sits upright. He has aged a month in five minutes.

"What's going on?" I am trapped in a mantra of fear.

"The needle went past the epidural region and into the spinal area." His eyes remain fixed on the monitor.

"And?"

"The spinal regionis much more sensitive to the painkiller. In effect, your wife suffered an overdose."

My ears burn. "What's the epinephrine do?"

"It counteracts the effects." The doctor removes his wire-rim glasses and rubs his brow. "I've only encountered this once before in fifteen years of practice." The spectacles return to his face. "Your wife is going to be alright, and your baby is in no danger." His hands clasp together tightly. "I'm very sorry." The threat of a lawsuit swirls about the room.

"It's okay," I say accepting his offer. "Francesca's father is a doctor. We understand."

"Thank God," is the unspoken reply.

Little hand halfway between four and five. Big hand obscures six. Four-thirty. My brain struggles to compute the difference between water breaking and now. Five. Six. Seven hours.

"Can you move anything?" I ask.

Francesca wiggles her right index finger.

The fetal monitor marks 10 PM with a squeal.

"Ready to push?" asks Yvette.

"Okay," dribbles out from underneath the oxygen mask.

"I'm going to ask you that question again," warns our guardian angel, "and this time you're going to give me an answer with attitude."

Francesca nods in agreement.

"Are you ready to push?"

"Ready." For the first time in hours, a familiar strength returns to Francesca's voice.

"Good girl!" Yvette offers her patient an ice chip. "When the contractions start to build, you push." The fetal monitor's contraction indicator races upward. "Push, girl, push."

Francesca grips the bed railing. Her jaw clenches shut. Her face turns crimson.

"You've got to push down here." Yvette points to the pelvic region. "You keep doing what you just did, and you'll pop a blood vessel."

The fetal monitor's blank ink line spikes sharply upward.

"Here comes the next one," I report dutifully.

"Don't you think I can *feel* it?" Francesca bears down, thrusts with all her might and then exhales.

"Close," Yvette leans over the bed. "But no cigar. You've got to push much longer. All you did was move the baby slightly forward and then back."

"Francesca, look at me. Open your eyes!" Her eyes flutter open, then shut.

"You're not breathing—you've got to breathe." Francesca exhales more evenly.

"Here it comes. Remember...short shallow breaths. Watch my fingers."

"Hee. Hee. Hee," she exhales.

"Relax your neck," advises Yvette, "You're still pushing in your face. Pretend you're making a bowel movement."

One AM. Is it possible?

Sixteen hours ago Dimas, the painter, wished us luck.

"Three centimeters," announces an orderly.

"The doctor wants to give you another hour before he considers a cesarean. You want to keep trying?"

"Yes," grunts Francesca.

"Good girl."

"C-section."

"An hour ago you said you didn't want one." Yvette lays a cold compress on Francesca's forehead.

"I know." Tears flow from my wife's eyes. "I changed my mind."

"You don't want a c-section. You've worked too hard."

"Shift change," announces Yvette. "Trish is going to take over."

"Please stay." Hours of perspiration have transformed Francesca's paper robe into a limp, transparent membrane.

"Trish is a friend of mine. You're in good hands."

A short, stout battle-ax clutches Francesca's hand. "Only you can push," counsels Trish. "Inhale deeply, hold it, and push."

Francesca's sweat drenched face glistens in the glow of glaring examination lights.

"You're about to have a baby." Doctor Newfeld wraps his hands in clear latex gloves. He stands at the base of the bed, framed by the dreaded squat bar. Assistants rush into the room and assume preordained positions at machines and probes.

"Push," spurs the doctor.

"Uhhhhh," hollers Francesca.

A face.

"Harder!"

Two arms.

A primitive, guttural groan leaps from Francesca's mouth. "Aaaaaah!"

Ten fingers.

"Keep it up!" urges Trish.

"Mmmmmah…"

Two feet.

"One more," urges the doctor.

"Eeeee-gah!"

A cry. A high pitched yelp.

"Do…you…want?" The LDR spins around me. "Cut…the…cord?" A male, pony-tailed nurse offers me scissors.

"Huh?" Time skips forward and back.

"It's a boy," someone announces.

"Eight pounds fifteen ounces," ricochets through my ears.

Two eyes open slowly.

They move left, then right. Left, then right.

"What's going on?" they demand. "What is this place?"

❖   ❖   ❖

From: pherman@—.com
To: Family and Friends
Cc:
Subject: EH IPO

(Hollywood) - Shares of Enrico Herman (EH) opened up sharply on positive news about his long-term growth prospects.

Initially priced at 7.0 lbs., EH opened at 8 lbs. 15 oz at 2:38 AM. Twelve leading investment houses have placed a "Strong Buy" recommendation on the stock.

"We expect Enrico's weight to increase consistently over the next ten years. We are recommending our clients purchase now," said Mark Katz, an analyst at Conglomerate Worldwide Investments.

EH co-founders Francesca Manarola and Perry Herman are very bullish on Enrico. "We plan to hold onto him indefinitely," said Perry.

Originally scheduled to go public on January 20th, EHpremiered fourteen days early due to intense investor interest.

Saint J—Hospital underwrote the offering.

❖   ❖   ❖

From: CousinN@—.com
To: pherman@—.com
Cc:
Subject: RE: EH IPO

As co-founder of a similar business with three similar investments, I absolutely agree with the decision to retain your investment indefinitely. Nevertheless, your business plan should take the following into account:

1. For the next twenty years your company will generate major expenses but no income. (Investment bankers refer to this as a "Loss Leader.")

2. In the beginning stages, your investment will develop a unique communication system totally incompatible with your current communication technology.

3. In the advanced stages, the investment will ignore any instructions issued by the board of directors. It will run itself for better or for worse. Often worse.

Love
Cousin N—

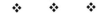

❖ 7 ❖

"The time has finally come to meet my maker."

I crane my head upward to find the source of the unexpected remark. Piled on top of a forgotten comforter rests the unsung hero of pregnancy, Mister Fluffy.

"What are you doing up there?" I ask.

"Waiting for the end," he replies morosely.

A step stool raises me up to Mister Fluffy's altitude. "Hi."

"I'm ready for the bin." The pink wonder falls into my arms.

"Not so fast," I protest.

"Don't mock me," he snaps. "It's bad enough already."

"Enrico needs a sister."

"He does?" A smile creeps across my compadre's cloth casing.

"Absolutely."

"A sister is a good thing." The down feathers relax.

"Looks like you'll have to hang around a while longer."

"Looks like I will."

Mister Fluffy wraps himself around my waist. "I knew you were a decent guy."

"Really?"

"Yeah, the moment I met you."

"Don't push your luck."

Mister Fluffy heeds the warning. "I thought you were kind of a shmuck."

"Better."

My Wife Is Pregnant

Acknowledgments

Thanks to my sister-in-law and Victoria Giraud for proofing the manuscript. I am also indebted to Dr. Janice Kinter, my therapist and personal Yoda, who helped rediscover the author in me. Finally, I want to thank Betty Peskin, my first fan.

End Notes

Information attributed to *The Merck Manual of Medical Information* appears in:

Berkow, Dr. Robert, Beers, Dr. Mark H., and Fletcher, Andrew J. The Merck Manual of Medical Information, Home Edition. (Whitehouse Station, N.J., Merck Research Laboratories, 1997), pp. 1157-1158.

Glucometer Elite® XL Diabetes Care System is manufactured by Bayer AG. Do not rely on the instructions described in this book when using the Glucometer Elite® XL. Consult a licensed physician about any issues regarding gestational diabetes. Bayer AG does not endorse or condone any activities or ideas described in this book.

About the Author

Perry Herman, father of a baby boy and husband to a busy executive, lives in Los Angeles. His eclectic background includes professional acting, comedy writing, journalism and computer programming. Perry was a cast member of *The National Lampoon Players'* live sketch comedy show and also performed at Los Angeles' renowned *ACME Comedy Theater*. His voice has been heard in many television and radio commercials including the acclaimed *Yo Quiero Taco Bell* chihuahua campaign. After scouring the bookshelves for a candid account of an expectant father's journey and finding only joke books and dry "How-To" manuals, Perry decided to write this book.

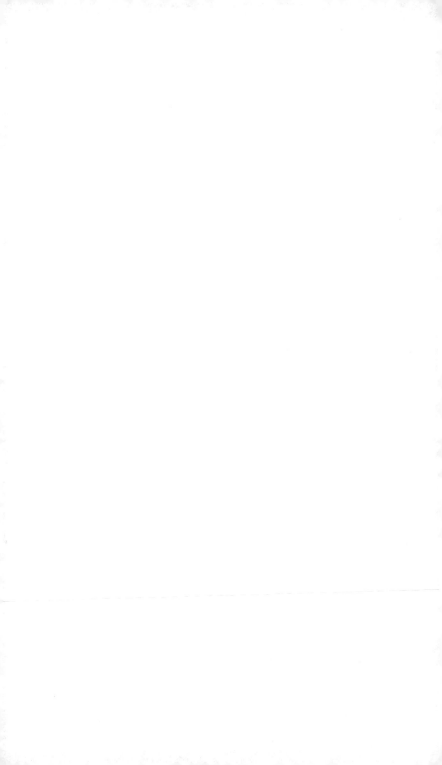

Made in the USA
Lexington, KY
16 December 2016